HESITANT HOPE

A memoir of anguish, endurance and healing

HELEN DEVRIES

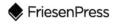

Suite 300 - 990 Fort St
Victoria, BC, V8V 3K2
Canada

www.friesenpress.com

Copyright © 2018 by Helen DeVries
First Edition — 2018

All rights reserved.

No part of this publication may be reproduced in any form, or by any means, electronic or mechanical, including photocopying, recording, or any information browsing, storage, or retrieval system, without permission in writing from FriesenPress.

ISBN
978-1-5255-2075-4 (Hardcover)
978-1-5255-2076-1 (Paperback)
978-1-5255-2077-8 (eBook)

1. BIOGRAPHY & AUTOBIOGRAPHY, PERSONAL MEMOIRS

Distributed to the trade by The Ingram Book Company

To my husband, Sid DeVries,
whose love and support gave me courage,

and

to the Medical Team,
whose knowledge and skill gave me a second chance.

TABLE OF CONTENTS

1 Remembrance Day 2013 1
2 Pathology Doesn't Lie 19
3 Choices 35
4 Christmas and Chemo 49
5 Folfox Encounter 65
6 One Day at a Time 81
7 Making the Cut 97
8 Surgery 111
9 Recovery 125
10 Reflecting on a New Beginning 145
Epilogue 167
Glossary 169
Acknowledgements 173

1

REMEMBRANCE DAY 2013

That mark our place; and in the sky
The larks, still bravely singing, fly...

—John McCrae, "In Flanders Fields"

"I'm very sorry we've had to meet, Mrs. DeVries." Dr. Vickie Martin, still clad in a colourful surgical cap and scrubs, has just entered my semi-private room at Kingston General Hospital followed by an entourage of doctors and students. She perches on the foot of my bed and folds her hands reverently in her lap. I'm momentarily stunned by the unusual conversation opener and stare at her in silence as she begins to explain what she found during my surgery. The left ovary, which appeared abnormally large on pre-op imaging, showed signs of disease and was removed. The right ovary was of normal size and appearance and remains.

Prior to surgery, a CT scan of the abdomen revealed a cloudy area on the lower right side that prevented any diagnostic conclusions. During surgery, the cloudy area was found to be concealing a tumour on the appendix. Dr. Jay Engel, a gastrointestinal surgeon, performed a bowel resection—a hemicolectomy in medical jargon—to remove the tumour, together with the appendix and a portion of the colon. The assumption going into surgery was that the diagnosis would be ovarian cancer, and for that reason Dr. Martin, a gynecological surgeon and oncologist, took charge of my case. The discovery of an appendix tumour, however, put that theory in doubt. The surgeons also discovered a substantial volume of mucinous material throughout the abdominal cavity and additional tumour growth on the abdominal wall.

"You don't think I have ovarian cancer?"

Dr. Martin chooses her words carefully.

"Until the pathology reports are in, we can't confirm the type of cancer or what stage it is."

The expression on her face tells me there's more. I can't believe this is happening. My throat is dry.

"There may be things you can't confirm without the pathology, but this is serious, isn't it?"

She nods solemnly. A lengthy silence ensues.

Dr. Martin slips off the end of my bed and takes my hand in both of hers.

"We're going to take very good care of you, Mrs. DeVries."

The medical team files from my room, leaving me with my family.

My husband, Sid, and I are enjoying a relaxing summer at United Empire Loyalist Park in Adolphustown, Ontario, where our RV is parked for the 2013 season. We spend our leisure walking in the seventy-two-acre park, cycling, or just sitting by the shore enjoying the activities of the local swan family.

Of late, the buttons on my jeans and capris have been getting harder to fasten. Perhaps I need to cut back on the burgers and beer. I've also noticed I don't have quite as much lung capacity when I'm cycling—the hills really make me puff. Trying to maintain a healthy weight is an ongoing challenge.

As the lazy, hazy days of August give way to September, I decide to stop procrastinating and pick up a FOBT kit from my doctor's office. All previous tests were clear, and I'm not worried about this one—just a precaution. About two weeks after returning the kit, however, I receive a call from Dr. Robinson, our family physician, telling me the test was positive for the presence of blood. She is scheduling me for a colonoscopy. Within a week, an envelope arrives in the mail from the Gastroenterology Clinic at Hotel Dieu Hospital confirming my appointment and providing detailed preparatory instructions for the procedure.

By mid-October, the RV has been delivered to storage for the winter months, and I'm excited to be returning to the city. While still snuggled between warm sheets on my first day back, I begin planning my day. The sun is streaming through our bedroom window, but no pleasant twitter of birds accompanies my waking moments as in the park.

When my mental "to do" list seems long enough, I breathe a sigh of satisfaction, letting my hands come to rest on my tummy after turning down the covers. My satisfied smile fades when I discover a lump on my left side. It feels surprisingly firm and about the size of a golf ball. The location is about where I imagine my left ovary should be, or perhaps a little higher. I get out of bed quickly still probing my belly, but once I'm standing the lump disappears. I continue with my day, stopping occasionally to check for the lump, feeling relieved when I fail to find it. Even a bedtime check produces nothing out of the ordinary.

I sleep well, but the first wakeful moment occurs simultaneously with my hand reaching toward my abdomen. There it is again.

"What time does the doctor's office open?"

I keep checking my watch.

Finally, at 8:30 a.m. I call. The medical receptionist doesn't hesitate when I tell her what I've found, booking me with the nurse practitioner later in the day.

When I arrive at the clinic, the nurse practitioner checks my abdomen then asks me to remain on the examining table while she leaves to confer with the doctor. Minutes later, she returns with Dr. Robinson. Pressing and probing, Dr. Robinson asks if *this* hurts or *that* hurts? After completing her examination, she tells me follow-up is in order and prepares a requisition for an ultrasound.

As soon as I get home, I call for an appointment at Kingston MRI Medical Clinic, only to find there's no opening for more than three weeks. Such a long time for this foreign presence to occupy my every thought without knowing its intention. I will touch it again and again, feeling the frightening firmness, praying it will be gone the next time I check.

"Come on, pull yourself together!"

My first prep day for the upcoming colonoscopy is October 29. It's a Tuesday, and my instructions are to take two Dulcolax tablets at 5 p.m. I reluctantly comply, resolving to enjoy my evening.

My morning begins early with a 5 a.m. trip to the bathroom, followed by several more at roughly half-hour intervals. At approximately 7:30 a.m., I develop abdominal cramping and the trips to the bathroom cease. The cramping continues unabated for several hours. By early afternoon, I'm running a fever and experiencing chills, so I place a call to Dr. Robinson's office and leave a message. When she returns my call a short time later, she advises me to go to the Emergency Department.

Although the last few weeks have raised some health concerns, stepping over the threshold of the emergency room is the beginning of the roller-coaster ride of my life. The reception area reveals the expected assemblage of distressed faces, some with hacking coughs, some with haphazard, blood-stained bandaging, and others whose ailments I can only guess. Certainly, the coughing makes one wonder whether you weren't better off suffering at home, but fortunately, the triage nurse, whose function it is to determine which patients need to move quickly to the next tier, soon leads me away to a curtained cubicle. After taking my temperature and checking my blood pressure and pulse, she turns to leave.

"A doctor will see you shortly."

The ER physician is a young man of medium height and build with short, curly, black hair and heavy black-framed glasses. His white coat looks fresh and clean, and I wonder if he just started his shift. He begins by introducing himself, then moves quickly to the questions. He wants to know what brought me to the Emergency and where it hurts. He wants me to describe the pain for him. I answer as best I can. After a brief examination, a CT scan is ordered and quickly completed.

While I wait for results, the sounds of the busy ER draw my attention. The young man with the blood-stained bandaging has been delivered to the cubicle next to mine. He needs to have a broken bone in his leg set, and based on the frequent moans there's no doubt he's in agony. After receiving medication for his pain, the moaning gradually subsides, and before long he's talking with considerable bravado about the details of his injury.

"The painkiller must be potent," I mutter to Sid, who's seated beside my stretcher.

"My guess is it's more likely an excess of alcohol talking," he whispers.

In a few moments, the doctor returns to discuss the findings of the CT scan. It shows a cloudy area over the appendix that makes it difficult to determine what's going on there, and the left ovary appears enlarged as expected. Because the pain is in the centre of my abdomen and I describe it as being similar to the onset of labour, the uterus is also of concern. The doctor says he has asked a general surgeon, who is in the operating room at the moment, to come and give his opinion on the likelihood of appendicitis.

We settle in to await the arrival of the general surgeon. Sid takes my hand and squeezes gently. I can see the worry on his face and the fear in his eyes. Because any medical concerns I've had in the past always turned out to be false alarms, I seem to be riding a comforting wave of denial at the moment in spite of suggestions to the contrary.

"I tried to call Sandy and Adam while you were having your scan, but neither of them were home. I left messages."

While waiting for my next examiner, double doors open across the room revealing two men in white coats guiding a stretcher. As they make their turn into the walkway at the foot of my cubicle, I notice the stretcher is completely sheeted from one end to the other even though it's obviously occupied. I drop my head back on the pillow and close my eyes. It's going to be a long night.

The general surgeon appears at about 10 p.m. After introductions, the familiar questioning begins again. "What brought you to the Emergency? Where is your pain? Describe your pain for me. Have you been sick to your stomach? Are you hungry?"

The answer to the last query is an obvious yes. Because I'd been prepping for a colonoscopy, my diet was clear fluids. Much to my disappointment, the question wasn't being asked out of concern for my empty stomach. The surgeon completes his assessment with a physical examination before taking his leave.

Once again, we resign ourselves to wait. The nurse peeks around my curtain to tell Sid there's a call for him at the desk.

"That was Sandy," he says on his return. "I've filled her in on what's happening, and she'll call her brother. Adam called her before she had a chance to listen to my message, saying he wasn't able to reach my cell phone and wondered if she knew what was going on."

The ER doctor returns to advise there is one more specialist he'd like to have evaluate my case before any decisions are made—a gynecologist.

Although my curtained cubicle keeps me blind to most of the activities in the busy examining area, my imagination is running amuck thanks to the unusual sounds. A new patient in the adjoining cubicle is creating a problem for his nurse.

"You need to lie down, sir." Her voice is loud—the firm tone of a woman accustomed to giving orders.

The man makes no audible reply.

"Stop spitting on the floor and lie down, please."

Over the next few minutes, the nurse repeatedly implores the man to stop spitting and lie down, receiving only the occasional grunt for her efforts. When two authoritative, male voices join the conversation, order is restored. I'm very curious about my new neighbour, but my imagination will have to suffice.

The gynecologist appears well after midnight. She is particularly interested in the location and description of my pain and examines the area thoroughly, all the while monitoring my comfort level. By this time, exhaustion has set in, and I'm finding it difficult to answer the doctor's questions. I feel muddled. I know I'm answering her, but I can't remember what I've just said. I hope I'm not causing confusion. Everyone seems confused enough as it is. When the ER doctor returns, he tells me I'm to be admitted. "I'm sorry you've had to wait so long, but we wanted to be sure we were admitting you to the right department. You'll be going to gynecology."

When we're alone again, Sid looks at his watch.

"I think I should go home for a bit," he says reluctantly. "The cat will be hungry, and maybe I can catch a few winks while they get you settled in your room." With a hug and a kiss, he's gone. I punch my pillow, pull up the blanket that's been keeping my feet warm, and close my eyes hoping I, too, might catch a few winks.

The next thing I know, a little lady hugging a clipboard is softly beckoning me from slumber. "I'm the admissions clerk," she chirps, "and as soon as we get your forms completed you'll be taken to your room."

Once again there are questions.

It's 5:15 a.m.

The short nap in the emergency room did little to relieve my exhaustion, and I continue to drift in and out for the next couple of hours. Sid discovers my new location around 7 a.m., and we exchange bits of conversation during my wakeful moments. A nurse arrives to check vitals and post an NPO notice over my bed. My housecoat, slippers, and toiletry kit are part of the care package Sid brought from home, so I take the opportunity to freshen up. I'll feel better, and the time and effort required will be a distraction from the absent breakfast tray.

It's mid-morning when a petite, young woman enters my room.

"Good morning, Mrs. DeVries. I'm Dr. Martin, and I'll be taking care of you. How are you feeling this morning?"

After introducing Dr. Martin to Sid, we begin discussing the events of the last twenty-four hours. Dr. Martin expresses her concern regarding the uncertainties presented by my symptoms and the CT scan and tells me x-rays and an ultrasound will be done this morning. She has also arranged to take me to the operating room this afternoon to obtain a biopsy of the uterus and conduct a more thorough pelvic examination under anesthesia.

Riding the calming wave of denial is becoming difficult. The possibility of a false alarm is fading with each procedure. The repeated reference to an enlarged ovary is hard to ignore, particularly when ovarian cancer has such a lethal reputation. But I mustn't jump to conclusions. Nothing is certain yet.

With the additional imaging completed, I wait nervously for my ride to the OR. The knowledge there will be no incision provides some relief, but I'm not looking forward to the anesthetic. I try to recall when I last had a general. It must have been the year after Adam was born, and we decided our family was complete. I remember feeling quite nauseous after that surgery.

The trip to the OR takes place in the early afternoon, and the next thing I remember I'm back in my room. Did the procedure answer any questions or did it create more?

When I see Dr. Martin again, she's attempting to mobilize a surgical team, hoping to take me back to the operating room. She's insisting a gastrointestinal surgeon be in attendance, so it appears she still isn't sure what else she will find in addition to the diseased ovary. At about 4:30 p.m., Dr. Martin concedes she has been unable to pull it together. There will be no immediate surgery.

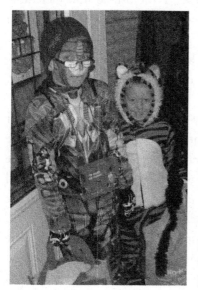

"The good news is, though, we're going to get you some dinner."

A morsel of cheer at the end of an otherwise anxious day.

In spite of the trauma playing out inside these walls, the city outside is celebrating. It's Halloween. The little ghosts and goblins are causing commotion in every neighbourhood. Doorbells are ringing, dogs are barking, and bowls of treats are being raided. I have just received a charming e-mail photo of two little trick-or-treaters, my grandsons. Six-year-old Samuel is a superhero, and three-year-old William is a tiger. This makes Grandma smile.

As the evening draws to a close, Sandy arrives to see for herself how I'm doing. She has lots of questions about how my day went, what we learned, and what will happen next. We don't have as many answers as she would like, but this is true for us as well. I'm lucky Sandy lives nearby. Hugs, kisses, and the comforting warmth of a loved one's hand at a time like this are beyond value.

The bustle of nurses and the clatter of breakfast trays mark the beginning of my day on November 1. Sid will arrive soon, and together we'll face another day. We've had our share of drama over the past forty-five years and somehow managed to emerge stronger and wiser. Now more than ever, I understand how incredibly fortunate I am to have such a devoted partner. I've taken so much for granted.

Shortly after the breakfast hour, Dr. Martin arrives, greeting us with a cheery, "Good morning! How are you feeling, Mrs. DeVries?"

She tells us she's booked my surgery for Monday, November 11, and expects it will take approximately three hours. If, as she expects, we are dealing with ovarian cancer, she will remove the uterus, both ovaries, and the omentum. An abdominal port will also be installed to receive chemotherapy once I'm healed. In the meantime, I am free to go home.

After changing from the hospital gown to the clothes I wore on Wednesday, I gather my things, slip into my jacket, and head to the exit. As I step through the revolving door, I'm greeted by cool, refreshing, autumn air. I close my eyes and breathe deeply, savouring the sensation. Exhaling slowly, I will the knowledge of the last two days to exit with my breath. I open my eyes—but my reality has not changed. I'm standing under the hospital portico waiting for Sid to pull up with the car. No words pass between us on the ride home, but when he reaches for my hand, the urgency in his grip speaks volumes.

As I step across the threshold of our apartment, a wave of emotion floods over me. The acknowledgement of what I likely carry with me, what I am bringing into this sacred cocoon is crushing me, breaking my heart. Sid's arms encircle me. I lay my head against his chest, sobbing uncontrollably. This is *not* how it's supposed to be. This is *not* the way we planned it.

The flood of tears finally easing, Sid reminds me that nothing has been confirmed yet, so we must do our best to soldier on in spite of the nagging uncertainties. I call the children to let them know I'm home and that surgery is scheduled for Monday, November 11. Sandy and her husband, Geoff, plan to stop in tomorrow. Adam and daughter-in-law, Isabelle, who live in Gatineau, Quebec, will also visit for the weekend. The boys want to bring me some of their Halloween candy. I also call the Kingston MRI Clinic to cancel the upcoming ultrasound.

Our plan to travel south in January for a winter getaway seems out of the question, so Sid begins the necessary phone calls and paperwork to cancel our reservations and medical insurance. While he's busy, I ponder the question of who should be told about my impending surgery. If we try to keep my health issue a secret, I have no doubt that sooner or later rumours will begin to circulate. I decide to prepare a list of family and friends we will keep informed via e-mail in preference to an out of control rumour mill.

Having the family visit over the weekend is a great diversion from our sobering thoughts. There are lots of hugs and words of encouragement. Sam and Will head for the cupboard where the toys and books are kept, and I know they will soon be asking, "Can we go to the pool?" I will watch from the sidelines this time. Later, they'll pass out the books and move from lap to lap as each is read. One sweet face is missing from this gathering, our granddaughter, Hailey, who is away at school in Ottawa.

My goals for the week are simple: eat well, stay active, and avoid infection. I'm still sore from the biopsy and exploratory examination, but hopefully that discomfort will disappear soon.

I receive an e-mail from Sandy on the morning of November 7.

Good morning!

Forty-three years ago today, we were given to each other. Love you!

How are you doing this morning? xoxoxo

What a lovely thought. I spend some time reminiscing before I respond.

Forty-three years ago—in some ways it seems like only yesterday, in others, a lifetime ago. A part of me would like to have the chance to do it all again—so young, so naive, so unprepared. But when I see the wonderful person you've become, one would be crazy to toy with perfection. I love you daughter, and I'm so glad you're mine. Happy, Happy Birthday!

I'm doing well this morning. Just got back from the laundry room—starting to plan what I'll put in my suitcase for next week. I feel a little better each day, which makes me happy. I wasn't looking forward to going into surgery feeling crappy. Nothing on the schedule for today, so don't have to go out unless I feel up to a short walk.

Hugs and kisses,
Mom

HESITANT HOPE

Pre-surgical screening takes place on Friday. We're almost there.

It's Monday morning, November 11. I've been fasting since midnight, so after showering and dressing I'm ready. At the hospital, I'm banded with an identification bracelet, given a hospital gown, a pair of compression stockings, a bag for my clothes, and asked to change. I'm taken by wheelchair to a waiting area where Sid, Adam, Sandy, and Geoff are gathered. Together, we wait to meet with the anesthetist who, when he arrives, confirms my identity both verbally and by checking my bracelet, then asks several questions related to my health, all of which had been asked during the pre-op screening. One wonders why it's necessary to answer these questions again, but I expect the intent is to prevent errors or omissions and provide assurance to both patient and hospital staff that everyone is on the same page. The anesthetist confirms I'm to have an epidural for pain control, which will be inserted in the operating room.

I'm taken to a large room with about six beds—the OR prep area. After transferring from the wheelchair to a bed, an IV line is inserted and a hydrating drip attached. Dr. Jay Engel, the gastrointestinal surgeon who will be assisting Dr. Martin, takes a moment to introduce himself. He's a tall, cheerful man whose presence inspires confidence.

One by one, the other occupied beds are wheeled from the room.

It's my turn.

My family walks with me as I'm wheeled into the hallway. Before reaching the operating room, we stop for a moment. I receive kisses, gentle squeezes, and encouraging words from each of my loved ones, and then their voices fade as I'm wheeled through the double doors.

"Don't worry, Mom. Everything will be OK," are the last words I hear.

It's the eleventh hour, of the eleventh day, of the eleventh month.

The operating room is already a hub of activity. With the use of a step stool, I transfer from the bed to a seated position on the side of the operating table. The epidural will be inserted while I'm in this position. I recognize the anesthetist who is perched on a stool at the head of the table, so I know he's not the one preparing for the procedure. The voice behind me is that of a young female, a student, I assume. Some freezing is applied to the spot where the needle will be inserted. A nurse instructs me to lean on her and make my back as round as I can—like a cat. I feel a jab.

"Ow!"

"Where did you feel that?" the voice behind me asks.

"To the left of my spine."

There is silence for a moment, then I feel another jab.

"Ow!"

"Where did you feel that?" she asks again.

"To the left of my spine."

After one more unsuccessful attempt, the anesthetist moves abruptly from his stool to the position behind me. In a matter of seconds and with no further protest from me, the procedure is complete. An instrument clatters to the floor as the anesthetist makes a noisy return to his stool, and the nurse helps me lie down. I feel sorry for the young lady whose day is not going well.

The lights and the sounds fade.

"You're in the recovery room, Mrs. DeVries."

I squint at the bright, overhead lights as I recognize the voice of Dr. Martin. She leans over me, speaking distinctly.

HESITANT HOPE

"Mrs. DeVries, I don't think you're alert enough yet for me to discuss the surgery with you. Would it be alright if I talk to your family first?"

I have difficulty opening my mouth. My lips and tongue feel thick and uncooperative.

"Yes, don't make them wait," I slur. "They'll want to know."

My family is waiting ... pacing ... flipping pages ... wondering about another coffee ... checking watches ... waiting ... waiting ... waiting. How much longer?

The optimistic one would be Adam. He keeps saying, "Everything is going to be okay. If they find a problem, they'll fix it." That's pretty much how he's experienced life—things are always fine in the end.

Finally, Dr. Martin appears from behind the ominous double doors. She motions them to an adjoining room—smaller, private, brightly decorated, a children's playroom. She closes the door. The tone of her voice sets the stage. This can't be good. Not one of them believes this can be good.

Dr. Martin describes for them the rarity of what she found. A mucinous cancer with tumours attached to one ovary, the appendix, and a portion of the bowel. Each of the affected parts was removed. The bulk of the mucus was removed as well, but the abdominal organs are coated with this substance that carries with it the seeds for additional tumours.

"She came through the surgery well. She'll be able to go home in a few days and will have a normal recovery."

"Is there's no silver lining?" Sid asks pleadingly.

"She will be able to go home. I'm sorry, there's nothing more I can do."

Quietly, deliberately, Dr. Martin leaves the room.

The children have never seen their father like this—devastated, broken, weeping.

"She's my childhood sweetheart … she's my life … my love … it should be me, not her …"

Sandy reaches out to him, comforting him as best she can through her tears.

Adam is crying convulsively, gasping for air. "Nothing we can do? *Nothing?*"

They're all hugging, sharing their grief, being there for each other.

"I remember seeing pain in Adam's and Dad's faces I'd never seen before," Sandy told me months later.

After an unknown amount of time, Dr. Martin returns.

"Would you like to see her now?"

Silence.

They wonder how. How will they manage to swallow their pain and smile?

"I haven't talked to her about the surgery yet, so you must be composed. Adam and Sandy, I want you to go together. I don't want you to talk about results, and you shouldn't stay longer than a couple of minutes."

I have no memory of the children visiting me in recovery, but they say I complained of cold hands, so each of them held a hand while I drifted.

"It seemed it would be impossible to put on a happy face, even for a few moments, but it was so good to see you. It turned out not to be too hard just to smile and tell you we loved you," Adam told me months later.

"It was possibly the most difficult thing I have ever done," is Sandy's recollection.

Then Sid is at my side. He takes my hand and kisses my forehead.

"You're doing great, Darling! I love you."

HESITANT HOPE

What would I have seen if I'd been alert enough to look into his eyes?

Once settled in my room and fully awake, my family joins me. Their expressions speak of love and relief at being able to lay eyes on me again. Their gentle hands reach out to me giving me strength—the strength I will need as I struggle to come to terms with my rewritten future.

2
PATHOLOGY DOESN'T LIE

I want to hide the truth.
I want to shelter you.
But with the beast inside,
There's nowhere we can hide.

—Imagine Dragons, "Demons"

Perhaps it's the sedation. Yes, that has to be it. I heard what Dr. Martin had to say, and I understand, but I'm composed. Where's the anguish, the anger, the resentment? I feel numb.

My eyes are misty. I'm fragile, both physically and mentally. I'm under attack. I have no defense.

My mind, however, clings to the thought that as long as the pathology reports are outstanding there is still hope—the chance for a silver lining.

Dr. Martin arranges for me to have a private room, no doubt feeling it appropriate for our family to have some privacy considering the devastating news we've received. In my new space, Adam hangs two hand-painted watercolours from my grandsons, and he also places a vase filled with flowers in every shade of pink you can imagine on my tray table. He will be leaving soon to return to Gatineau. I will miss him.

When Sandy comes to visit after her workday is finished at the Napanee hospital, her first impulse is to clean everything within my reach with disinfecting wipes. She's aware of the risk of MRSA, methicillin-resistant Staphylococcus aureus, in healthcare settings and instructs me to insist that everyone entering my room either wash their hands with soap and water or use hand sanitizer. She encourages me to use the alcohol-based hand cleaner and also asks me to avoid touching my face where bacteria can easily enter the body through mouth, nose, or eyes. Unfortunately, I have a very itchy rash around my nose and mouth that is likely an allergic reaction to the rubber-like material on the rim of the breathing mask used during surgery or the gas delivered by it, so I'm failing to keep my hands away from my face.

Within a couple of days, the rash on my face fades, but I've developed an itchiness over my entire body. I'm certain a warm shower would be comforting, but I'm told this can't happen until the epidural is removed. The removal is done on Wednesday morning, and I wait expectantly for the promised assistance with showering. The itch is driving me crazy. I push my buzzer, only to be told the RNA is on her coffee break. I try reading to pass the time but have difficulty concentrating. Between the itch and being on new pain meds to compensate for the lack of the epidural medication, I'm extremely uncomfortable. I press the buzzer again. This time it's lunch break. I groan in frustration. Relax ... relax .... Another excruciating hour ticks by. When I buzz again, I've lost all patience.

"May I *please* have my shower now?"

Within minutes, a nurse appears with towels over her arm, and I'm soon finding the relief I crave amid the warm, soothing droplets. I'm not proud of my demanding behaviour, but it seemed my only option. The nurse tells me the itchiness is likely a reaction to the medication delivered by the epidural.

HESITANT HOPE

An e-mail from Adam helps me ignore the remainder of my allergic reaction.

Hey Mom,

I'm leaving work, headed to the airport for my trip to Toronto. Thought I'd send a little note because I'm not sure when you might feel like talking. I heard you had a pretty busy day. How's it going with the new pain meds? I love you lots, Mom. I can't wait to see you again this weekend.
Adam

Throughout the week, I have regular visits from both Dr. Martin and Dr. Engel. They are keeping a close watch on my incision, which runs from three centimetres above my navel to the edge of my pelvic bone. Surprisingly, there is no dressing over the incision, and it appears to be healing well.

I don't ask a lot of questions on these rounds. What's the point? Until the pathology reports are in, the answers will be vague. I'm not interested in vague.

As the week passes, the doctors become more interested in my bowel function. I learn I won't be released until I either have a bowel movement or pass gas. Dr. Martin is no modest violet and seems to relish popping into my room with a cheery, "Any farts yet?"

The week is winding down. I've passed the time with deep-breathing exercises to ward off pneumonia, ankle-flexing movements to aid circulation, and treks along the hallway arm in arm with Sid to regain muscle tone and balance. Several visits highlighted my week. My sister Betty Ann and her husband, Arden, a pastor, spent some time and offered prayers for my recovery. Sisters-in-law Jane and Jo also visited, and cousin Lloyd and Sue came bearing a graceful calla lily. I've read, I've examined the courtyard from my window numerous times, sipped copious amounts of liquid, and slept a great deal. If only I could …

Mission accomplished! I'm going home. It's Friday, November 15.

I'm happy to be leaving the hospital. Although everyone is very kind, it would be difficult to imagine wanting to stay once one is on the road to recovery. Going home under the circumstances, however, is far from joyful. I will have the comfort of familiar surroundings and the lavish care of family and friends, but what will I look forward to? Certainly, to spending as much time as possible with my children and grandchildren. Sid and I will make plans for tomorrow, next week, and probably even next month, but next year? I will celebrate my sixty-fourth birthday soon. Will it be my last? It would be a darn shame if I never collect my monthly dues from Prime Minister Harper.

The lavish care begins with Sid purchasing a smoothie machine and preparing a variety of nutritious and delicious liquid treats that sit well on my fussy tummy. Sandy arrives on Saturday with homemade cookies and vanilla-flavoured protein powder to give the smoothies an added boost. She also spoils me with a soothing manicure and pedicure. Adam is able to visit again, and after preparing a delicious, roasted-chicken dinner, concocts a savoury stockpot that will provide tasty soups in the week ahead. With such professional pampering, I should be completely healed and reenergized in no time.

I'm having a weepy weekend. Sandy and Adam are with me, and Hailey is breaking away from her hectic study schedule to visit as well. I'm fearful I won't be able to control my emotions when Hailey arrives, but when she hugs me, the pleasure of her presence seems to outweigh my sadness. There is nothing that means more than having my loved ones near at this very frightening time.

My sadness is bound to my vision that when my body can no longer continue, my spirit will be freed to travel to another dimension. In my imagination, I see my spirit beginning its journey, drifting away from my mortal home. I can still see my loved ones gathered there, sharing a meal, talking, remembering, receiving comfort and strength from each other. The path I am on seems solitary. They have each other. I am alone. I don't want to go. I don't want to be separated from them. I don't want to lose them!

When our weekend guests depart, all is quiet again, and I'm content to spend plenty of time resting. I'm still taking hydromorphone, an opioid pain medication prescribed for moderate to severe pain, but, hopefully, I'll be able to switch to Tylenol without difficulty by the time I've taken the last dose.

We see the nurse practitioner at Dr. Robinson's office for staple removal on Wednesday, and I'm relieved to find the procedure almost painless. Sid is keen to assist when an extra pair of hands is needed to ensure that no staples have been able to escape detection in my navel. Because he must watch helplessly from a distance much of the time, it's a welcome boost for his psyche. The decision is made to leave a couple of staples at both the top and bottom of my incision—more healing is required. Upon returning two days later, however, some post-surgery fluid is still evident at both locations requiring the application of small dressings after the remaining staples are removed. An antibiotic is prescribed to avoid infection.

Two weeks have passed since my surgery, and my patience is wearing thin. Why haven't I heard from Dr. Martin? Surely the pathology reports are available by now. A call to her office reveals that some reports *are* available while others are outstanding and may require an additional week. While I'm trying to decide whether I'm disappointed or relieved, there's a knock. I open the door to find a neighbour and friend holding a plate of homemade muffins. I've known Marilyn since we made the move to apartment living in October 2012.

"Marilyn, it's so nice to see you. Please come in."

By September of 2012, a For Sale sign had been on our twenty-four hundred square foot home with acreage south of Napanee for two years. Many would-be buyers, particularly those from the city, are fearful of wells, septic tanks, and sump pumps, and few folks know what they'd do with the sixteen acres—not quite big enough for a hobby farm and not nearly small enough for mowing. Others are overwhelmed by the sheer size of our flower beds and vegetable garden.

The work involved in maintaining our home and property has always been a labour of love, but these days *labour* seems to be the key word. Sid's knees are painful, and arthritis in my spine is slowing *me* down. With Sid's help, I have already reduced the size of the largest bed by half, but it's still too much for me to manage. A decision was made to exchange our labour intensive lifestyle for one that would give us choices about how we spend our time and energy.

Miraculously, in the last week of September, the perfect buyer makes an offer. Closing date will be October 15. We have our work cut out for us. Before the end of the week, we've found our new home—a two-bedroom apartment on the twelfth floor at 1066 King Street West in Kingston. Little do we realize what a blessing it will be to live less than five kilometres from Kingston General Hospital.

HESITANT HOPE

Friends and relatives ask if we miss our flower beds, vegetable garden, and wide open spaces both inside and out, but the truth is we don't. We cherish the memories we've made, but we were ready for a change, a new adventure. We are delighted with our view of Lake Ontario, Lake Ontario Park, and the Cataraqui Golf & Country Club, and we appreciate the compact, efficient design of our eleven hundred square feet.

While picking up our mail in the lobby, one of the first neighbours I meet is a short, cheerful lady in a hot-pink baseball cap. As is so often the case, her name immediately escapes me minutes after we introduce ourselves, but I see her again, complete with the florescent baseball cap, when I attend an aqua-fit class in the pool.

One Friday afternoon at an informal gathering in the common room known as Happy Hour, I introduce myself to a friendly lady with a noticeably tidy hairstyle. Before long, I realize this is the lady in the pink baseball cap now sporting a becoming wig. Marilyn asks if my husband and I plan to travel south this winter. She and her husband, Bob, were in the habit of spending three months in Florida, but will be staying home this year. She was diagnosed with ovarian cancer in the spring and has just finished her first round of chemotherapy. Her attitude is so positive and her personality so vibrant, I can hardly believe my ears when she tells me she's seventy-nine years old—sixty-nine maybe. Over the next year, we pass the time of day whenever we meet, but after my surgery in November 2013, she is the first in the building to drop in for a few minutes with homemade muffins and words of encouragement.

"Be happy—cancer hates happy!" is Marilyn's mantra.

Another week idles by. The living room resembles a flower shop. There have been a number of deliveries as well as guests bearing gifts. Some visitors arrived with appetizing treats. Betty Ann spent several days baking her annual Christmas fare of loaves, squares, cookies, and chocolate-dipped delights, and then she delivered a generous portion of each conveniently packaged and ready for the freezer. No one will miss out on homemade goodies at our house for the next month. Marion, a longtime friend now living in Ancaster, arrived with an edible arrangement almost too beautiful to touch.

There are only three days left in November. We awoke this morning to a breathtaking sight—a continuous blanket of white as far as the eye can see, dotted with billowing, alabaster, cotton candy on stalks of chocolate bark among evergreens partially iced with ivory cream. As the morning sun rises over the cityscape, its rays flirt shamelessly with the diamond-encrusted snowflakes creating a dazzling display. What a wondrous world this is!

The lengthy wait for pathology results is becoming tedious. In spite of my need to know the dreaded details of my serious situation, I still allow myself frequent daydreams of denial. My friend Heather says she believes it's really the luxury of hope I'm creating for myself because we can never know for sure what path our lives will take.

The telephone finally rings on Tuesday morning, December 3. I take the kitchen phone, Sid picks up in the office.

"Hi, Mrs. DeVries, it's Dr. Martin. How are you doing?"

"I've been very weak, but I think I feel a little stronger."

"I see improvements every day," Sid pipes in.

"Your voice sounds better I think."

"Yes, others have said that."

"I presented you yesterday at the gastrointestinal tumour rounds and then again this morning to the gynecology group. Dr. Engel was at rounds yesterday, and the final pathology is confirming that it is a tumour, a cancer, of the appendix, and that the ovary is a metastatic implant, we would call it. There is a lymph node that is involved within the block Dr. Engel removed. There's only *one* lymph node of eighteen that is involved, and the margins of the colon that Dr. Engel cut away are clear. Of course, there are lymph nodes that remained after surgery because they were not resectable based on their location. We knew there would be an issue of needing to have chemotherapy regardless.

"Cancers are staged, with the maximum stage being stage IV, and this is a stage IV. The metastatic implants on the ovary are from the same type of cell as the appendix—it is not a separate tumour. So one of the medical oncologists who treat gastrointestinal cancers is going to see you. There are three of them, and they are all very, very lovely, Dr. Booth, Dr. Hammad, and Dr. Biagi. I think you will find any one of them very approachable. I know them all personally, and they are wonderful, wonderful, and I mean that very sincerely."

"Dr. Engel is no longer involved?"

"No, Dr. Engel is a surgeon exclusively, and my specialty is gynecology, so I'm putting a consult in for you to see one of them, but I don't know which one it will be. There was a discussion about a CT scan just as a baseline from the surgery, but I think it's a bit early to organize that because of the surgical issues. There's still going to be a lot of inflammation, so oncology can determine the timing of that, and they will also arrange a consultation with the Toronto team for discussion of your case. You will likely go there after you make contact with the team here."

"Do you have any idea how long it will be before I see the oncologist? Will it be after Christmas?"

"No, no, it will be before that. Usually, they will see you within two weeks. Again, they're still going to need you to do some healing. Let me know when you get your appointment, and I will come down to see you for a post-op check if I possibly can, if I'm not in surgery.

A long silence.

"Helen?"

"Yes, I'm still here," I managed through my tears.

"Sid, she needs a hug. Okay, Sweetie, you take care, and I'll be in touch."

Stage IV—definitely *not* what we wanted to hear. After that pronouncement, nothing else registered.

Every scrap of hope has been exhausted. Every fingernail clinging to the ledge of denial, shattered. Now I'm falling ... falling ... falling. There is, indeed, no silver lining.

The well of tears seems bottomless. My vision of drifting away, leaving the ones I love, is consuming me. Something about this suffering is familiar: when our first born arrived prematurely, unable to survive; when my father died; when I learned my mother had breast cancer and would soon die; when my sister Evelyn died. The well was deep on those occasions, too.

Sid and I spend much of the afternoon in each other's arms. I willingly absorb the comforting warmth of his body. His slow, rhythmic breathing soothes my broken heart. His strong, meticulous heartbeat insists it isn't over. Life—one heartbeat at a time.

We make the necessary calls to Sandy, Adam, and Betty Ann. Sandy and Geoff come over after their workday ends. Before bed, I send a short e-mail.

Dear Family and Friends,

I spoke with the doctor today, and it was confirmed that the primary tumour was the one in the appendix. I'm being referred to an oncologist who deals with gastrointestinal cancers, and I expect to be seen within the next week or two. He will be able to provide more information about my particular type of tumour and offer treatment

options. The news was pretty much what we expected, not pleasant, and most unwelcome.
Helen

A new day begins with a lovely surprise delivered by the postman—a birthday card from Hailey. This card is *exclusively* from her—a unique marker of her first year away from home. It includes a Starbucks gift card.

Hi Hailey,
Thank you for the lovely birthday card! I'm looking forward to a stop at Starbucks.
Your Mom and Geoff were here for dinner last night. We ordered pizza because I hadn't had any since before the surgery. It was good.
I guess you'll be preparing for exams at this point. Eat healthy, get enough rest, and be confident. I know you will do well!
Hugs & Kisses
Grandma

Dear Grandma,
You are most welcome!
Starbucks is liking me lately. The combination of finals approaching and the cold weather has been drawing me there, maybe a little too often. I have my first final on Saturday, biology, then three others by the 16th. I've been studying my buns off these past few days. I went out and bought a cart full of fruit today because your little

message about eating well made me think about how much junk I've consumed lately.

I hope you've continued to heal since I last saw you and that you're feeling much better.
See you at Christmas! :)
Hailey xoxoxox

A call from the secretary at the office of Dr. James Biagi comes on Friday morning. I will see him on Wednesday, December 11. Birthday flowers are delivered from my niece Debbie and her family, and on Saturday, December 7, my birthday, Betty Ann and her daughter Angie visit, bringing flowers. I haven't seen Angie for several months, so it's a special pleasure—such a thoughtful, sensitive soul. The handwritten message in her card reads:

Dearest Aunt Helen: Wishing you a birthday filled with happiness and celebration for the wonderful life you've lived and the graceful way you've met, and continue to meet, challenges head on with class and dignity. In celebration of beautiful you, happy 64th birthday!
Much Love & Many Prayers, Angie xoxo

Adam and Isabelle arrive in the afternoon with Samuel and William. Little William has been in the habit of running at top speed to deliver his hello hug, but after being cautioned about Grandma's sore tummy is reluctant. I wish I could turn back the clock—I do miss those enthusiastic hugs. Samuel is concerned about what was removed during surgery, but he smiles happily when I tell him they only took the parts I don't use any more.

Eight of us gather at Milestones for a birthday luncheon on Sunday. It's a happy get together thanks to Sam and Will who keep everyone smiling and laughing with their light-hearted chatter. Too soon, it's time to part. Back to jobs and classrooms, except for Adam who has arranged to stay with us for an extra day. Sweet!

The Cancer Centre of Southeastern Ontario is a modern facility in the Burr Wing at Kingston General Hospital. After parking in the area designated for cancer patients, we enter the bright, spacious lobby and scan for an elevator. Much to my surprise, the first thing to catch my attention is a polished grand piano. The elevator to the other three floors is to our right, together with a number of wheelchairs. We take the elevator up one level and find ourselves at the entrance to the Chemotherapy Unit where we're directed to the Cancer Centre reception desk on the other side of the open lobby area.

After checking in, a volunteer guides me to one of two computer terminals in the waiting area and shows me how to complete a questionnaire that evaluates the severity of nine symptoms common to cancer patients: pain, tiredness, nausea, depression, anxiety, drowsiness, appetite, wellbeing, and shortness of breath, on a scale of 1 to 10. When finished, a printout is delivered that I'm to give to the nurse once summoned to the examining room. This procedure is to be repeated at the beginning of each visit.

The reception area is large and busy. Some wait to have blood taken in the lab, while others wait to see their doctor. My name is called, and we're greeted by Dr. Biagi's nurse, Lou. She checks my weight, reviews my history, and questions me about how I'm feeling today. When her note taking is complete, she leaves, and we wait nervously for the doctor.

After introductions, Dr. Biagi confirms the information I've already been given from the pathology report and advises that because this cancer is rare there is no protocol for treatment at KGH. He tells us about a treatment available at Mount Sinai Hospital in Toronto called HIPEC surgery. He describes it as surgery at a "whole new level" that requires a lengthy and difficult recovery.

"It offers the possibility of a cure."

Stage IV cancer diagnosis ... possibility of a *cure*. How does this compute? My mind is spinning in an endless loop. I should question him, but I don't.

"I'm sixty-four years old. I've had a good life. This doesn't sound like a desirable option for me at this stage."

"Nonetheless, I'm going to set up a referral for you to see Dr. Andrea McCart at Princess Margaret Cancer Centre in Toronto, and I hope you will listen to what she has to say."

"Yes, of course I will listen, but if I choose not to have this surgery, what can I expect?"

"You will likely have three to six months of symptom-free living. Once you become symptomatic, I would like to see you, and we will start chemotherapy to help control your symptoms. The overall outlook I would say is likely two and a half to three years, maybe a little more, but certainly not five years."

Well, there we have it. No beating around the bush, just the facts. The future of a cancer patient with mucinous appendiceal adenocarcinoma.

3
CHOICES

*You don't get to choose how you're going to die. Or when.
You can only decide how you're going to live. Now.*

—Joan Baez, *Daybreak*

"If they think I'm going to let them turn the rest of my days into a schedule of medical appointments, they can just think again. I've *seen* what happens to people who choose regimes of chemotherapy and radiation, and I won't let them do that to me. Why would anyone choose nausea and vomiting over normal living just for the sake of a few more weeks or months? Enjoy the good days you have left, I say. We *all* have to go sooner or later."

Sid is sitting beside me on the sofa, eyes downcast, making no reply. I don't know what he's thinking and I'm not going to ask. This has to be my decision.

I should be uncomfortable with this choice, not to seek his counsel. It's been our habit to discuss matters of significance, and I could always count on his objective opinion. But not this time. What I *can* count on is his unconditional love and his understanding of my need to figure this one out on my own.

Looking around the apartment we've so recently established together, the solution to our desire to have more fun and leisure in our lives, I can't help wondering who will be sharing this dream with him five years from now. When I was biopsied for breast cancer in my late thirties, jealousy reared its head, and my mind raced with thoughts of him in a new relationship. But with this new threat, I find myself hoping he'll have someone to share the good *and* the bad with. I wouldn't like to think of him alone should illness strike. How would I have endured these last two months without him? Even the inevitable ravages of old age are better shared, we've already discovered.

There are things I definitely won't miss. Pet peeves, things I've never learned to take with the proverbial grain of salt, never been able to get past or let go of, even after all these years.

But what about the things I *will* miss? Sid and I will mark our fiftieth wedding anniversary on April 20, 2018. I would like to share that day with him. We enjoyed a tour of The Netherlands and Belgium on the occasion of our fortieth, and it would be such fun to plan another trip to Europe, maybe a river cruise.

Hailey and Scott have been dating for three years. Perhaps there will be a wedding after college graduation—two delightful celebrations to share

Samuel and William have *so* much growing to do. I would like to continue watching the changes each year brings. Samuel has a genetic eye disorder, Leber congenital amaurosis, that causes serious vision loss. Encouraging research is underway that could provide him with improved vision in the future. Wouldn't *that* be a thrill to witness!

I pick up my iPad and open the Google search engine.

For the next week, I scour reputable websites for information about my type of appendix cancer and HIPEC surgery, HIPEC being an acronym for Hyperthermic Intraperitoneal Chemotherapy. Appendix cancers account for only 0.5 percent of all intestinal cancers. Only about 20 percent of these are shown to be mucinous adenocarcinomas, although the most recent research suggests the percentage is rising. Because appendix cancer is rare, extensive and dependable statistics about the success of treatment and life expectancy are not available. The limited information that can be found should not be the basis one stakes one's life on.

Our family Christmas celebration is planned for Saturday, December 21, at Adam and Isabelle's home in Gatineau. We plan to travel on Friday, giving us Saturday as a backup in case the weather is bad. A phone call from Dr. Biagi's office, however, has us adjusting our schedule. An appointment with Dr. McCart is set for Friday at 11:30 a.m. Unfortunately, the weather forecast for *both* Friday and Saturday threatens freezing rain, so we decide it best to drive to Toronto on Thursday afternoon and stay in a hotel near the hospital.

What should I wear for the lengthy trip? I need an outfit that won't put pressure on my incision, particularly at the waistline. My garment of choice for the past few weeks, a nightgown, is not an option. Most of my wardrobe consists of slacks and skirts, so I decide to go shopping for a shift or shirt-style dress.

When I enter the dress shop, I'm greeted by a friendly sales clerk.

"I'm looking for a loose-fitting, medium-weight dress with half or three-quarter length sleeves," I tell her. "I've recently had abdominal surgery and can't tolerate anything tight at the waist. Would you mind picking a few pieces you think might work while I rest a bit?"

After showing me to a dressing room, she begins her search.

A few minutes later, she returns with three outfits. "Will you be alright, or may I help?"

"Thank you, I'll call if I need you."

Taking a few moments to review the possibilities, I choose the silky, black dress with an attractive pattern of thin, white, horizontal stripes to slightly above the knee where the stripes alter to varying widths and sparkle in shades of lime and fuchsia. I set about the demanding task of changing. The air in this confining space is warm and stale, and my skin begins to glow from the effort. I slip the dress over my head, satisfied to see how easily it drops over my curves, no tugging or adjusting required. The deeply scooped neckline eliminates the need for a troublesome back zipper and showcases my favourite necklace. The sleeves fall slightly above my elbow, and I tie a narrow, matching belt loosely at my waist. This is the one—casual, comfortable *and* chic!

"I hope your surgery was a success and you'll be feeling stronger soon," the sales clerk offers as she carefully folds my dress.

"They removed a tumour—malignant. I'm not sure where I go from here," I reply matter-of-factly.

"Oh, I'm so sorry. That must be just terrible for you."

"It certainly wasn't pleasant news, and it's taken me a while to get my head around it, but the fact is, we're *all* going to die. I just happen to have a little more information than the average person about the timing and circumstance."

She looks at me, uncertain at first. "I guess you're right. I never thought about it that way."

I thank her for being so helpful and leave the store, resolving to be less candid with the next stranger I encounter.

When Sandy shares my diagnosis with her co-workers at Lennox and Addington County General Hospital, she receives a flood of sympathy and support. She also learns, to her amazement, that one of the staff members has an aunt who has had HIPEC surgery for an abdominal cancer similar to mine. Johanne lives in Quebec City, and according to the staffer is doing well.

My reaction to this news is a mixture of surprise, disbelief, and hopefulness. To have already found someone who shares my rare diagnosis is surprising, particularly when most of the medical community are baffled. "Appendix cancer? I've never heard of it."

Could she *really* be doing well? Oh how I would love to believe that. There's only one way to find out.

Hi Johanne,

My daughter, Sandy Johnson, who works at the Napanee Hospital with an acquaintance of yours, gave me your name and contact information. She told me she believes you've had the same kind of surgery I'm considering, and that you would be willing to share your experience with me.

I was diagnosed with mucinous appendiceal adenocarcinoma in November following surgery to remove the primary tumour of the appendix and one ovary where metastatic implants of the primary tumour cells were found.

I have an appointment in Toronto on Friday to meet with Dr. McCart. The following is a link to the Mount Sinai Hospital website that explains a bit about her procedure.

http://www.mshfoundation.ca/Page.aspx?pid=1575

Following my appointment, my husband, Sid, and I will be travelling to our son's in Gatineau, Quebec, for our family Christmas. It's a very busy time of year with all the festivities, but I look forward to hearing from you when you can find the time to write.
Wishing you and yours a happy, healthy Christmas!
Helen DeVries

Within minutes of sending my e-mail, the telephone rings. It's Johanne, her voice friendly and cheerful. Our exchange is immediately comfortable as we speak freely of the appalling turn our lives have taken. Upon hearing Johanne's use of the epithet "jelly-belly," referring to the buildup of mucous in the abdomen, it's clear to me our diagnoses are a match. She tells me about her surgery in May 2012 at a Montreal hospital, confirming that the recovery is indeed long and difficult—she was unable to manage on her own for the first six weeks. She now has a drain because of disease in her liver, and she admits that for her surgery was not a cure. A follow-up surgery was offered, but she declined. In spite of her prognosis, she believes her first operation was worthwhile and encourages me to give it every consideration.

Was it a mistake for me to talk to Johanne?

The drive to Toronto on Thursday is refreshing. The massaging warmth of the sun through the windshield and the ever-changing scenery are doing wonders for my spirits. Arriving at the hotel, I find our pristine suite a pleasure to behold: no half-empty glass of water on the night table beside a prescription bottle; no well-worn housecoat and slippers waiting expectantly at the foot of the bed; no scissors, gauze, and tape on the bathroom vanity in case my incision springs a leak again; only beautiful, tidy normalcy. After enjoying our comfortable quarters for a time, we walk to a nearby restaurant for dinner. There is little tension about tomorrow. We savour our choices from the menu and enjoy the ambiance of a flickering fire in the nearby hearth.

When you stand at the intersection of University Avenue and Gerard Street West, you are surrounded by hospitals—Princess Margaret, Mount Sinai, Toronto General, and Sick Kids. It's an impressive sight. We find our way to the door of Princess Margaret after paying twenty-five dollars for parking. Memo to file: Don't complain about parking fees in Kingston.

The lobby is huge, and the frenzied activity reminds me of an airport terminal. There's a busy deli to our right, a bank of glassed-in elevators to our left, a patient library straight ahead, as well as an information kiosk and plenty of seating. The ceiling of this area rises several stories. On the statuesque brick wall to the left, giant cursive letters proclaim:

"Believe It. We Will Conquer Cancer In Our Lifetime!"

We take the elevator to the Gastrointestinal Clinic on the 4th floor.

Between my appointment time of 11:30 a.m. and 1:30 p.m., I'm interviewed by the receptionist, a nurse, and Dr. McCart's assistant.

"Hello, Mrs. DeVries, I'm Dr. Scheer. I work with Dr. McCart. I'd like to talk to you about why you've come to see us and what we may be able to do for you. After that, Dr. McCart will see you. Do you have any questions before we begin?"

"Yes. Could you please explain my diagnosis in more detail? I don't feel I know much about it."

"Tell me what you know."

"I know I have mucinous appendiceal adenocarcinoma, and I know it's stage IV."

"Well, I would say you know quite a bit. Besides staging, cancers are also graded as low, moderate, or high, based on how the cells compare with normal tissue. Grading is usually an indicator of how quickly the cancer is likely to grow and spread. Your appendix cancer is a particularly rare moderate grade. We usually see high grade or low grade. When we see a low-grade tumour, it's a very slow-growing, indolent tumour that produces jelly or mucin. These tumours are like a jelly doughnut, and the mucin is squeezed out or leaks out and eventually fills the abdominal cavity. When you have a high-grade appendix tumour, it acts more like a colon cancer, a solid tumour. It likes to spread, go to the lymph nodes and get into the bloodstream. When you have a moderate-grade tumour, we don't really know *which* way that tumour wants to go. In fact, your tumour is showing signs of wanting to go in both directions. It's showing us the mucin, the low-grade component, and then you also had a positive lymph node which is more what a colon cancer would do, the high-grade component.

"So what's the bigger problem? The bigger problem is the colon cancer behaviour, the solid component of the tumour, not the mucin. The mucin is a problem because it can build up, and we can talk about what we can do about that, but what's going to *get* you is if this tumour decides to spread and get into the bloodstream and into the liver and into the lungs, just like it already started to go to the lymph node. So that's the part we're more concerned about. From that point of view, I believe Dr. McCart will recommend starting off with chemotherapy, getting a toxin into the bloodstream to kill any little cells that are thinking of setting up shop, because right now there's no sign that it has spread anywhere else.

"You've already had a very good surgery. Dr. Engel and Dr. Martin removed the primary source of the disease, and they've given a good assessment of the disease that they saw. Now we need to deal with the disease that we *can't* see. Because your tumour is the unusual intermediate grade, however, there are no guidelines. There are guidelines for high grade and low grade, but with intermediate grade we're in a no-man's land, so we're making this up as we go."

"How encouraging!" I quip. "Does this mean I may become one or the other?"

"No, it just means your tumour has features of both. As I was saying, I believe Dr. McCart will recommend we start with chemotherapy, a full cycle of six months at two-week intervals with Folfox. You will need to have a full work up of CT scans of the chest, abdomen, and pelvis so we have a baseline of what we're starting with. It's been about six weeks since your surgery, so we could get the baseline CT scans done in early January, and then you could start chemotherapy. These scans would be repeated at three months and again at the end. We'll compare all of those scans, and if the disease remains stable with no evidence of additional disease popping up in other places, then we can talk about the big surgery we do here to deal with the disease that's in your abdomen. The report provided by Dr. Martin indicates they saw a lot of mucin in the pelvis."

"Did they remove all of that?"

"They removed what they could see by suctioning it out. That doesn't mean there wasn't a fine coating that remained on the organs and abdominal wall. They saw some small nodules on the large and small intestines.

"If everything looks good on your CT scans after chemotherapy, then we would do a laparoscopy, which allows us to have a look inside your abdomen with a camera. That will help us determine just how much disease there is and whether or not we think we can remove it all with the surgery.

"It's a little bit too early to talk about the big operation because we don't know what the trajectory of your disease is at this point. I'm hopeful it's going to stay that intermediate to low grade, but if it takes a turn in the other direction and all of a sudden we see a deposit in the liver or the lungs, which I don't expect, that would change our direction. I don't think that's the way we're going, but I can't say for sure. So I can't give you a lot of information as to what the plan is other than we do recommend chemotherapy, and we do want to see you again. We think there's a reasonable chance that if you want to, we will end up at surgery."

"The CT scans and the chemotherapy, would that take place in Kingston?" Sid asks.

"Yes, Dr. McCart will contact Dr. Biagi to let him know our plan, and he will let her know what's going on in terms of updates from you. If your CT scans remain stable, we will coordinate for you to see us again."

"Dr. Biagi said that if I chose not to consider your surgery, he wouldn't start chemotherapy until I was more symptomatic, perhaps early summer."

"Yes. If you said, 'Listen, thanks very much, but that surgery sounds ridiculous,' and it is, a twenty-plus hour operation with an incision from your breast bone to your pelvic bone because we need to remove everything that's in your abdomen. We remove all of the disease that we can see, and it usually ends up being a piece of colon, the uterus, the ovaries, a little bit of this, a little bit of that, a little bit of a whole bunch of things. Then we fill the belly up with heated chemotherapy and flush that through for a while. You'll be in the ICU for a couple of days and in hospital for two to three weeks. It's a big deal, but it's the *only* option to go for a cure. We're not saying that it's necessarily an option. It might not be. So if you said, 'No way, I don't care, I'm not going for it!' then there would be no point in giving you chemotherapy. We would keep our tricks until there was a problem. But if you said, 'Yes, I'd like the option,' then I think we should go ahead with chemotherapy. Let's say you don't have chemotherapy, you've already had disease that's spread to a lymph node, so presumably there's disease in the system. It may not be. It may have been all that was there, but if you don't have chemotherapy you're leaving yourself open to it popping up somewhere else."

"I think I'd like to keep my options open. How am I likely to respond to this Folfox? Some people seem to sail through chemo with little difficulty, while others . . ."

"This is not like breast cancer chemotherapy—you don't lose your hair. Dr. Biagi will be better at describing this because it's his specialty. The biggest side effect is numbness and tingling in the finger tips, but nausea is not a huge component. Folfox is better tolerated than many others.

"May I examine your abdomen?"
"Of course."
"How is your health otherwise?"
"I have arthritis in the upper part of my spine that creates a lot of discomfort."
"Any heart or lung problems?"
"No."
"Is there a family history of colon cancer?"
"No."
"Have you had a full colonoscopy?"
"No."
"You *do* need a full colonoscopy. I'm going to have a few words with Dr. McCart, and we'll return."

Wow! A deer in the headlights—that's me. The small examining room is crowded with speech balloons floating placidly about: particularly rare moderate grade ... positive lymph node ... full six-month cycle of Folfox ... no guidelines ... the big operation ... laparoscopy ... unknown trajectory ... twenty-plus hours ... remove everything in your abdomen ... go for a cure ... it might not be ... keep our tricks."

I peer frantically through the balloons for Sid—another deer in the headlights.

"Mrs. DeVries? I'm Dr. McCart. Dr. Scheer has been filling you in on some details about your appendix cancer. Your cancer is a particularly rare moderate grade, and for that reason I'm recommending chemotherapy before surgery. You need to have a baseline CT scan before chemotherapy begins and another one when you're finished. Unless something shows up on the CT scan that would suggest surgery wasn't feasible, then we would plan to do the operation once you've had time to recover from the chemotherapy.

"Dr. Biagi said you weren't sure about the operation, and you don't need to decide right now. I'm going to give you my booklet to take home and read. It's going to tell you maybe more than you want to know, but it's what you need to know if you're having the operation. It will tell you all the possible things we could do and all the possible complications. Most of the time, there are no complications, but just so you know. Now the other thing you should know is that chemotherapy alone won't get rid of this cancer forever—surgery might. That's why we would put you through all of this."

"I find it difficult to comprehend the possibility of a cure."

"Yes, it *is* possible, but it's not a guarantee."

"I understand."

"I wouldn't put people through my operations without the possibility of getting rid of their cancer. Even if it doesn't get rid of it forever, what it does do is prolong the time it takes for it to come back. There definitely is benefit either way."

"I've read a bit about the surgery, and initially I just shook my head. But when I consider what my options are, it sounds like short-term pain for long-term gain."

"Right, right, that's it exactly. Appendix cancer is a spectrum. The grade is very important for how we think about it. With the low grade, you can have the chemotherapy, then the operation, and go away and have nothing for ten years, whereas if it's high grade, it can be back causing you problems within a year. You're in the middle somewhere, and it's hard to know where you fall. We're being on the more aggressive side—we might not need to be—but we're trying to get on top of it."

Sid asks for confirmation. "So she would get chemotherapy for six months followed by a recovery period, then we'd be coming back to see you, and you would decide, based on CT scans and a laparoscopy, what would happen next?"

"Yes, and the decision—beside you deciding yes or no—is whether anything shows up outside the abdomen. As long as it stays in the abdomen and we determine it's removable, then we would go ahead with the surgery."

"If the surgery is an option, when would it likely take place?"

"You would finish chemotherapy in June and have a month to recover, so we would likely schedule for August or September."

"I have a question. I brought in my list of medications, and one of the prescriptions I've been using is an Estring. It helps control vaginal atrophy and problems with urinary tract infections. Can I continue to use it, or is my cancer estrogen sensitive?"

"You can continue to use it, not a problem in this case.

"So if you decide you want the surgery to be an option, call Dr. Biagi's office and tell him you want to go ahead with the chemotherapy. Any other questions?"

"No, but I'm sure I'll have lots the next time we meet."

"Are you driving back today?"

"Yes, we are."

"Drive carefully—its none too pleasant out there."

We hurry from the hospital around 2:30 p.m., anxious to leave the city behind before rush hour wreaks havoc. A light rain is falling, but, thankfully, the temperature is still above freezing. With the appointment behind us, we are focused on returning home to make final preparations for our trip to Gatineau. I'm determined to put my medical issue on the back burner and enjoy our family time over the next few days. Of course, everyone will be anxious to hear about my appointment, and I will be glad to share my feeling that a ray of hope has begun to flicker at the end of my long, dark tunnel.

You'd think I already had enough information to absorb for one day, but as we leave the city my curiosity gets the better of me, and

I pick up Dr. McCart's patient education booklet. *Cytoreductive Surgery with HIPEC (Hyperthermic Intraperitoneal Chemotherapy).*

I turn to the first page.

4
CHRISTMAS AND CHEMO

*Life isn't about waiting for the storm to pass.
It's about learning to dance in the rain.*

—Anonymous

The weather is being uncooperative. The last leg of our trip yesterday was frustratingly slow due to a drop in the temperature that turned light rain to a hazardous freeze. Saturday morning finds us white-knuckling our way to Gatineau under similar conditions. Normally, Sid would refuse to venture out in such brutal circumstances, but I suspect he's choosing to push the boundaries of prudence because he knows how important it is for me to be with our family on this special occasion.

By the time we'd arrived home from Toronto, I had worked my way through Dr. McCart's booklet. The seventeen pages covered definitions, surgical criteria, pre-surgery, surgical overview, post-surgery, hospital stay, and release information. For *this,* I will keep my options open by subjecting myself to six months of chemotherapy? It feels like one nightmare after another. This makes the surgery I had last month look like child's play.

The anxiety created by our treacherous drive on ice-slicked highways is akin to the distress I feel when I consider what I'll have to endure to give myself a chance to live a few more years: to be open from ribcage to pubic bone for possibly twenty hours or more, to have every organ removed and examined inch by inch, to have nodule after nodule plucked from sensitive tissue, to have some organs completely excised, others partially, then the heated chemotherapy wash for ninety minutes that will sear every surface it touches. I'm glad we'll soon arrive in Gatineau where the joy of the season and the cheerful commotion of excited children will send my morbid thoughts running for cover in the hidden recesses of my brain.

In spite of the risk, we arrive safely after three and a half hours, one hour more than our usual time. A thick cover of fresh snow, towering pines, and colourful lights framing the roof line above amber-lit windows make Adam and Isabelle's home as inviting as any pastoral Christmas card scene. Near the front entrance, a jolly inflated Santa Claus and sledding Mickey Mouse bob about in the chilling wind entertaining us as we approach.

When we open the door, shouts of "Grandma! Grandpa!" greet us, together with the spicy scent of mulled cider. Samuel and William each take a hand and guide us to the Christmas tree, proudly pointing out ornaments they contributed, as well as laying claim to the artful decorating. Ten bright but very flat stockings at the fireplace will soon be bulging with treats and surprises.

Vignettes of Christmases past flash before me:

My father and I are trudging through knee-deep, blowing snow on our way to the woods. It's never easy convincing him of the need for a Christmas tree, but eventually he tires of my pestering just in the nick of time. He carries an axe over his shoulder, and I carry a bow saw over mine.

HESITANT HOPE

Our six-week-old baby girl is mesmerized by the Christmas tree that's been twinkling at the living room window since the first week of December. Beneath its boughs, small, brightly-wrapped packages await little hands. She'll need our help this year.

The Christmas tree is backdrop for a very special photo. My frail and ailing mother is seated in the rocking chair, a tiny baby swaddled with lacy white in her arms. Her first great-grandchild. The next photo will show four generations with Betty Ann and her daughter Crystal included. Mother will not see another great-grandchild, nor will she see another Christmas.

Adam's voice and the mouth-watering aroma of roasted turkey and stuffing wafting from the kitchen call me back.

"How did your appointment with the specialist go, Mom?"

"It went well I think. I learned quite a bit about appendix cancer and the only option for treatment. Dr. McCart thinks that with six months of chemotherapy followed by her radical surgery, I could be looking at the possibility of a cure, or at the very least, a substantially longer lifespan."

"Wow, that's great news!"

"It definitely puts a different slant on things. After the surgery in Kingston, I didn't think I had a future. Now, I feel there's hope, if only I can deal with my fear of the procedures and the uncertainties of the outcome. Dr. McCart gave me a booklet to read about her surgery. It's pretty graphic. I'd rather not go that route, but the other option provides no hope at all."

"So, you're not sure?"

"I'm still thinking it through, but no matter which way I look at it there seems to be only one logical conclusion, so perhaps I *have* made up my mind. I just need to give it a bit more time."

"I'm so glad there's something they can do."

I may not wish to let the opinions of my loved ones affect my decision to accept or refuse treatment, but there's no question where they stand. How foolish to believe their desires won't be woven into the fabric of my choice.

Our traditional Christmas dinner is a sumptuous delight as usual. For the first time ever, I was unable to prepare the "my Mother makes the world's best pie" pies, but Sandy, who has become a pie-maker extraordinaire herself, did the honours in my place. She has also perfected a crockpot stuffing that is not only delicious, but saves the last-minute digging to relieve the bird of its tasty treasure.

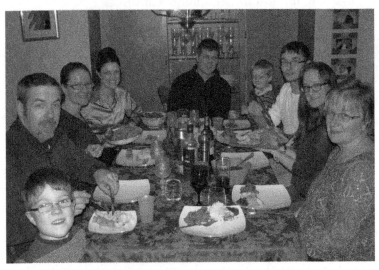

Left to right: Sam, Geoff, Sandy, Isabelle, Adam, William, Scott, Hailey, Helen. Photo by Sid.

After dinner is over and the table is cleared, Sam and Will produce one of their many games and chant, "Qui est là? Qui est là? Who wants to play Qui est là?"

If you've never experienced eight adults, in addition to two children, sitting around a table communicating in the language of barnyard animals, you don't know what you're missing! Being able to remember who made which sound and which animals are on the cards lying face-down on the table when they are briefly turned, will allow you to collect the most cards and win the game. A roaring good time, or more accurately, a barking, clucking, and mooing good time is had by all.

For the last few years, we've been drawing names and placing a dollar-value limit on purchases so gift-giving could be less of a focal point, the children excepted, of course. This Christmas, however, some are ignoring the guidelines with me being the beneficiary. Adam had drawn my name for this year, and his gift is a duo of gift certificates, one for the Kingston Grand Theatre and the other for the nearby Windmills Restaurant. Sandy's surprise gift is a lovely set of silver mother-daughter rings which are intricately carved with symbols from nature—trees, wind, moon and stars. I feel very special.

Gifts become a sensitive matter when combined with grave illness. I remember unwrapping a birthday gift from my mother some four months before her passing. It was a simple gift, a pair of kitchen towels, but knowing it was the last birthday gift she would ever choose for me was heartrending.

The unwrapping is followed by excited sharing of new treasures and much reading of instructions to aid in the construction and mastery of new toys. Sam and Will are particularly enamoured of remotely-controlled race cars from Aunt Sandy and Uncle Geoff. Sunday brunch is being prepared in the kitchen, and mouths are watering—the coffee and juice that started our day are a distant memory to growling tummies. Another meal fit for a king.

Gathered around the table, we talk of plans for the remainder of the holiday season. There will be more feasting with other family members, and outdoor sports are high on the priority list of most given the abundance of snow.

Christmas Day celebrations wouldn't be complete without a walk in the snow and the odd snowball taking flight. The boys enjoy their toboggan on the slopes in the backyard where Dad has begun piling snow for a giant slide. Before the afternoon sun fades, we gather our belongings and bid fond farewells. It's a fine day for travel.

Although Adam and Isabelle gave us their bedroom on the main floor so stair-climbing wouldn't add to my fatigue, I'm nevertheless very tired and glad to lie back and relax for most of the trip home. Inescapably, my thoughts return to the urgency of my situation and the decision I must make. Even though I'm terrified of the procedures laid before me, does it make sense to turn my back on the possibilities? If I do, the cancer will likely begin to cause discomfort within the next six to eight months, then palliative care would begin. I don't like that terminology—care of the seriously ill with a view to relieving discomfort. There's no doubt it has its place—*I just don't want to be in that place!* I'll call Dr. Biagi's office tomorrow.

On Monday, January 6, 2014, I'm at the KGH Cancer Centre completing another questionnaire. I've learned it's referred to as ESAS (Edmonton Symptom Assessment Survey). My appointment with Dr. Biagi is for 1:45 p.m. In the days leading up to this appointment, I've read and reread Dr. McCart's patient handbook. Some points will require clarification at our next meeting, but it seems as I become more familiar with the details of the surgery, my fear is morphing into determination and commitment.

"This is what I need to do."

I've started distancing myself from my body, thinking about it more as a possession, a luxury automobile perhaps, valuable, useful, attractive, and worth taking care of. If my car has a problem, do I fear letting a reputable professional work on it, or do I simply deliver it to the best garage in town and trust the mechanic to do what he is trained to do?

Dr. Biagi opens the door of the examining room where Sid and I have been waiting.

"Hello, Mrs. DeVries, Mr. DeVries. I got your message."

"I know when we last talked I left you with the impression I wasn't interested in treatment, but after my appointment in Toronto with Dr. McCart and much soul-searching, I've decided to take the first step toward the HIPEC surgery, which is a six-month cycle of chemotherapy.

"Of course. In order to give this type of chemotherapy, it's important that we establish a special intravenous access that's more long-lasting than the drip you're used to around the time of surgery. It's called a PICC line, peripherally inserted central catheter. Are you familiar with that?"

"I noticed people in the waiting room at Dr. McCart's office with a stretchy, gauze sleeve on their upper arm, and I assumed it was related to an access for chemotherapy."

"We can show you what it looks like. It's a fairly simple procedure done in the Radiology Department, and the line would stay in place for the entire six-month period. It can be associated with some discomfort. Occasionally, it gets infected during that time period or causes a blood clot. You'd know there was a problem because your arm would swell and begin aching, and that's a reason to come in and have it looked at.

"If you're a swimmer and that's how you stay fit, this wouldn't be a good thing. You are able to shower with it wearing a sleeve, but we don't want it under water. If you're an avid swimmer, we could install a port under the skin, but it's not typically what we aim for because that's more of a surgical procedure."

"I've started to use the pool again since my incision healed, but I'm not devoted to it. I can do other things to stay fit."

"Good. The chemotherapy we will use is called Folfox. It's actually a set of three chemotherapy drugs, two of which are given over a couple of hours in the chemotherapy room here. The third, in a small bottle, is attached to your PICC line and carried home with you in a pouch belted to your waist. This drug will continue to infuse over the next two days, and then a nurse will come to your home to disconnect the bottle and flush the line.

"Then the question is, how well are you going to tolerate this? Is chemotherapy going to go well or not? We never know from one person to the next. I can treat the fittest young person, give them the same treatment I would give you, and you tolerate it better. There's no way of predicting. Usually, Folfox is fairly well tolerated for the six-month period, but occasionally we make people sick, so we need you to be familiar with the possible side effects, and the list is long. You're not likely to have all of them, but you need to know before anything happens so you won't be too concerned. Let's say you are treated on Monday, the bottle would come off Wednesday afternoon, and now you're at risk of side effects over the next couple of days. By the weekend, you should be feeling just fine. If you're not feeling well for the majority of the two-week period, we need to make adjustments. So part of the job here over the next six months is to keep you well.

"Some of the common side effects are upset stomach, sores in your mouth, numbness and tingling in hands and feet, watery eyes, changes to your skin, possibly diarrhea or just as likely constipation because of some of the medications we give to help protect the stomach. Occasionally, patients on Folfox lose all their hair, but that's very unusual. You're more likely to notice some thinning as time passes. Fatigue can grow over time. Very rarely, treatment can actually cause chest pain, and that's absolutely serious, so you need to be seen right away. Don't wait.

Chemotherapy also lowers the immune system, which puts you at risk of infection.

"So there's a slightly queasy stomach once every two weeks, then there's nausea and vomiting for four days straight, the extreme. It could be anything in between. The extreme is a concern because dehydration can occur, especially if you're not eating or drinking."

"If the symptoms were extreme, does that mean the medication needs to be adjusted?"

"Correct. It usually means we'll give a brief break from treatment until you recover, and when we continue we'll adjust the treatment accordingly."

"How do you monitor whether my kidneys or liver are being adversely affected?"

"Every two weeks, just before your treatment, I require a blood test that checks how your liver and kidneys are doing, and your immune system—is it down or is it okay? My nurse, Lou, and I have you in and check you over, assess how you're doing, and discuss how the last two weeks have been. Our care goes beyond that. Being a chemotherapy patient, we will educate you as well to call us with problems. Say you were still nauseous later in the week, you can call Lou and say, 'What can I do about this?' You can call us nights and weekends, so you've always got access to a chemotherapy specialist, a doctor, sometimes me. If you get a fever on Saturday, we don't want you waiting until Monday to call. We want you to help us keep you safe. These crisis situations are uncommon, but as long as you know we want you to call. I know this is a lot of information to take in all at once, so we'll provide you with paper copies of what we've covered.

"We need to make arrangements for insertion of the PICC line. Are you right or left-handed?"

"I'm right-handed."

"They'll try to use your left arm. When the catheter isn't in use, it just folds up against your arm. I'll also arrange for you to have a colonoscopy, and if it's clear, then you're done for five years."

I manage not to laugh, but this strikes me as humorous given I won't likely live that long.

"It isn't something you should have done while you're on chemo with your immune system going up and down, putting you at risk of bleeding and infection, so I'll arrange that right away. We will do a base line CT scan before we begin and halfway through your six months of chemotherapy. Hopefully, that scan will show a reduction in cancer tissue. Then, as we're finishing up another three months of treatment, we would do a final scan. Lou and I will make all these arrangements, and you will hear from us. I'll keep Dr. McCart up-to-date. Did you meet her?"

"Yes, I did. She was pleased with the detailed report you forwarded, and she was also very happy with the type of surgery that was done for my situation."

"Good."

"They were very complimentary," Sid adds.

"Well that's nice. I didn't ask her to do that."

The humour is a welcome break from an otherwise sobering conversation.

"I didn't suspect you did," I responded.

"Well, I think that's it. We've got a lot of work to do, and we're going to get started. Is that all right?"

"That's alright. My brain says this is what we're going to do. The rest of me is dragging along behind, but the brain is willing."

"Good, and our job is to keep you well. We'll make sure you know how to get in touch with us, and we'll be seeing you regularly."

"Sounds good."

"If you will sign this consent for the insertion of the PICC line, we'll let you go."

HESITANT HOPE

I am beginning to wear the weight of my commitment. Plans need to be made for moving forward on this lengthy and demanding journey. The first action I take is to call my dentist and request an early appointment for cleaning and a checkup before chemotherapy begins, since bleeding and inflamed tissue might prevent dental work over the next several months. Sid and I discuss the new pressures that will bear down on him as I begin to experience nausea and weakness. He is confident he can manage whatever is required, but I insist that with the added responsibilities of grocery shopping and food preparation as well as laundry, cleaning should definitely not be something he has to worry about. He agrees to give a half-day a week of housekeeping a try, and I contact Jessie, an experienced and caring worker who is also a resident in our building. She will come from 1 to 4 p.m. every Wednesday afternoon to clean, giving Sid a chance to be out without worrying about me. Many thoughtful, concerned ladies in the building have offered to spend time with me whenever needed, in particular, Emmy, a dear friend on our floor who checks in regularly, often delivering freshly baked treats and always asking whether there is anything she can do.

Appointment details begin to clutter our calendar. The colonoscopy on Friday, January 17, is the first to be penciled in; on Tuesday, January 21, PICC line insertion; Wednesday, Saint Elizabeth nurse and CT scan; Thursday, chemo seminar; Monday, January 27, lab and Dr. Biagi; Tuesday, chemotherapy. All the ducks are in a row.

Thinking back to the chain of events which took place during the last week of October when I was preparing for the initial colonoscopy, I have a gut-wrenching dread of those first two pills that begin the prep process. Logic tells me a repetition of the pain, fever, and chills that sent me to Emergency on that occasion is impossible because the conditions that caused the problem no longer exist. Still, it's with great trepidation that I swallow the pills. All goes smoothly, however, and on Friday morning the procedure is completed under the supervision of Dr. Robertson at Hotel Dieu Hospital with only a mild sedative, little discomfort, and very good results.

The following Tuesday morning finds me waiting nervously in the Radiology Department at KGH. The radiologist who will do my procedure introduces himself, then a friendly nurse confirms my identity, explains what will take place, and leads me into the operating theatre where she helps me onto the table. The site on my left upper arm where the line will be inserted is sterilized and injected with a local anesthetic. I wait, alone, in the chilly, darkened room for the freezing to take affect and the procedure to begin. A slender tube will be inserted into the large vein returning blood to my heart, then threaded upward until the leading end arrives in my chest just above my heart. This will be confirmed by x-ray. The exiting end, after being attached to a catheter, will be folded against my arm in the bandaging process. Before the arm is wrapped, a clear adhesive dressing will be applied to the entrance point to protect against infection.

I'm trying to be brave, but truth be told, the thought of having the tender tissue on the inside of my upper arm slashed deeply enough for the main vein to be fished out, with me awake, is horrifying. Telling myself that many procedures are done through the veins these days doesn't serve to calm the sickening wave rising from my gut. Why couldn't they just put me under?

"You'd better buck up kid … this is just the beginning."

The procedure takes only ten to fifteen minutes. I feel no discomfort until the freezing is out, but for the rest of the week I require meds to dull the pain.

I'm not sure how I feel about this intruder demanding direct access to my bloodstream and my heart. Despite the benefit of not being jabbed with a needle several times during each of the twelve chemotherapy cycles, it will be a constant reminder that my life has spun out of control, that I am no longer in charge. I should think of it as a helpful friend, but I doubt that's going to happen.

Brenda, a nurse from Saint Elizabeth Home Care, arrives on Wednesday morning. The visit takes about an hour and includes a medical history review, patient assessment, ordering of medical supplies, flushing the PICC line, and redressing the area. I'm pleased to see individually-sealed, moist swabs on a stick, looking very much like a lollipop, are used to clean the skin and the tubing at the insertion site. The nurse uses three of these sterile swabs, wiping only once with each side. My confidence in the care of the intruder is growing, and my fear of infection subsides slightly. As she's leaving, Brenda cautions me to expect a side effect commonly referred to as chemo brain. Apparently, I can expect to see a decline in brain function. This is not something I'm pleased to hear, and I decide I'll take a wait-and-see attitude rather than accept the information as gospel.

Wednesday afternoon finds me seated in the cafeteria at KGH. Minutes ago, I checked in at the reception desk in the Imaging Department reporting for my first CT scan. I'm given a large, plastic glass, complete with lid and straw, and told to drink a quarter of the contents over each of the next four fifteen-minute intervals. The content appears to be water, but has a distinct metallic taste. I'm envious of others seated around me with their bottles of juice or cups of tea or coffee and make little effort to hide my displeasure with each sip. Perhaps sitting in the cafeteria isn't a good idea. Will this elixir make me more photogenic? I should have asked. After the hour is up, I report back to Imaging where four scans are completed. My PICC line is used for the first time to inject dye into my bloodstream prior to the last two scans.

Sandy and Geoff join us for dinner on Thursday, then spend the evening in the kitchen making a variety of healthy snacks for me to nibble on when I'm receiving chemotherapy.

Sid and I are seated in a large conference room at the Cancer Centre with a dozen others on the afternoon of Friday, January 24. Some are cancer patients about to embark on a common journey, and the others are supportive spouses, family members, or friends. It provides some comfort to see I won't be alone while feeling my way through the frightening maze of cancer treatment. The seminar, called Chemotherapy and You, is led by a registered nurse trained specifically to work with chemotherapy patients. Some of the information is familiar because I've been reading the material provided by Dr. Biagi, but it's good to have it reinforced, complete with a PowerPoint presentation and detailed handouts.

The week ends on a celebratory note. Emmy's husband, Joe, has reached his eightieth birthday, and together with several other couples in the building, we've been invited to a cocktail party in his honour. Once again, I'm privileged to be in a supportive circle of friends whose good wishes provide encouragement.

My PICC line is used for the second time on Monday morning. Blood is being drawn for tests that will determine my suitability to receive the first chemo treatment. Since there are no drugs in my system as yet, the results should be normal. My blood is being drawn in the Chemotherapy Unit rather than the lab because the nurses there are familiar with PICC line procedures and have the necessary supplies at hand.

Now it's time to see Dr. Biagi, and Lou prepares me by checking my weight and asking how I feel.

"As I indicated on my questionnaire, my anxiety level is high. The thought of what will take place tomorrow and the uncertainty of how it will affect me is very stressful."

"The most difficult treatments are the first and the last," Lou advises.

"The last?" I question.

"Yes, by the time you get to the last one, your body is just so tired."

I don't understand. Shouldn't there be delight or at least relief associated with the last treatment? Guess I'll find out when I get there. I just want to have the first one behind me.

Dr. Biagi conducts a physical examination of my abdomen, listens to my lungs, and checks for swelling of the lymph nodes in my neck. My blood work is satisfactory, so an order will be placed with the hospital pharmacy where the drugs will be prepared for my appointment in the Chemotherapy Unit tomorrow morning. Some of our conversation seems geared toward determining my intention to follow through with the plan in place. I wonder what percentage of patients make a last-minute decision to abort? Before I leave, Lou gives me a wallet-size card that I'm to present at the Emergency Department should I run a fever of thirty-eight degrees Celsius for more than an hour. The card identifies me as a chemotherapy patient on Folfox.

Since my visit with Dr. McCart, I've been trying to deal with the depressing reality of *twelve* chemotherapy treatments. Six long months and twelve infusions of toxins designed to kill. Toxins that are not yet targeted to kill only cancer cells—they will kill healthy-dividing cells with the same rabidity as cancer cells. I write a column of descending numbers from 12 to 1 on a sheet of paper and attach it to the refrigerator door.

Tomorrow I will make the first mark.

5
FOLFOX ENCOUNTER

Look well therefore to this day;
Such is the salutation to the ever-new dawn!

—Kalidasa, "Look to this Day"

One last look in the mirror. The shapeless, grey top screams back at me—too many washings—but the sleeve is wide enough to allow access to the intruder. "Henceforth, thou shalt be dubbed Chemo Shirt."

The face staring back at me is stern, the lips set in a firm line, the eyes focused and determined. She seems to know what she's doing. If only I felt as confident as she looks. I check my purse for the necessary paperwork.

The air has a familiar January chill, the lake frozen as far as the eye can see, a solitary ice-fisherman the only distraction on an otherwise pristine snowscape. While Sid retrieves a discounted receipt from the Park & Pay kiosk, I pull a bright pink parking pass from the stapled bundle in my purse and place it on the dash. Reduced parking fees in the designated Cancer Centre parking areas is one of the perks of being a cancer patient, provided, of course, there is an available space.

Sid takes my arm as we pick our way across the snow-packed parking lot. For this appointment, we're entering the Cancer Centre from the George Street entrance instead of the main entrance on King Street West because I insist I'm quite able to walk from the parking area rather than be chauffeured to the front door.

The large L-shaped desk in the reception area holds a bowl of candy and a floral arrangement left over from Christmas. The receptionist reaches for the appointment sheet clutched in my hand while talking on the telephone and plucking away at her computer keyboard. After crossing my name off her lengthy patient list, she tells me to take a seat then disappears through the double doors near her desk with my paperwork. Before she returns, a nurse calls for the next patient from the same doorway.

There's commotion at the far end of the room. Belongings are gathered from the floor, and wheelchair brakes are released. A group of three passes. An obviously fatigued cancer patient slumps slightly forward in her wheelchair, her head wrapped in a colourful bandana. A disheveled, elderly man is guiding the chair, and a much younger woman carries purses, tote bags, and various pieces of clothing. They are greeted by the nurse, and the doors close behind them.

Among those remaining, a student, college-age, seated cross-legged while poring over textbooks, earbuds in place; a middle-aged man dressed in workmen's clothing; a well-dressed older couple, both looking well—I wonder which one is the patient?

"Helen DeVries." A nurse is waiting at the door, file in hand. "This way, please."

She leads us to a quiet corner with a window overlooking the lake. The room is large and bright. The usual hospital curtains hang from ceiling tracks. Several treatment stations line the wall, each equipped with a large leather recliner, small cupboard with countertop, IV pole, TV, and companion's chair.

HESITANT HOPE

As I settle myself in the recliner, a volunteer asks what I'd like to drink. My drink of choice, ginger ale, is delivered as the nurse squeezes two white, five-sided pills into my hand from individually wrapped packets—dexamethasone. The purpose of this steroidal drug is to stop the nausea and vomiting that may occur with chemotherapy. This medication should be taken with food, and it's only a few minutes before the volunteer offers me a packet of two Dad's Oatmeal Cookies.

My nurse disappears while I'm snacking, but soon returns with a clear plastic bag from the hospital pharmacy filled with the liquid medications I'll receive intravenously over the next two hours. She holds each pouch before me asking for confirmation that the information on the pharmacy labels is correct. Each bag is clearly marked with my name and date of birth. The pouches include Leucovorin, a faint yellow solution the purpose of which is to increase the activity of the anti-cancer drugs; Fluorouracil, a colourless solution used for treating cancer; and Oxalipatin, the third drug in the Folfox cocktail.

After donning rubber gloves, my nurse hangs the fluid pouches from hooks on the IV pole. The Leucovorin delivery line is the first to be passed through the computerized device on the pole, which she programs to control how quickly the solution will pass into my body.

Am I ready for this? How will it make me feel? I remember the patient in the wheelchair. How tired and ill she looked. Will that soon be me? No, Dr. Biagi said the goal is to keep me well, remember? I try to divert my thoughts. The tote bag we brought contains homemade snacks, iPad, a novel, and the morning newspaper. Sid will do the sudoku, and I, the crossword puzzle.

Minutes tick by. I watch the bag for evidence of a reduction in content and the line for signs of movement. I'm aware of tightening in the muscle tissue in my head similar to what you might feel at the onset of a stress headache. I recline my chair and try to relax. The volunteer stops by again, this time to ask if I'd like a warm blanket. It's obvious volunteers play an important role at the Cancer Centre.

After a half hour, the Leucovorin bag is empty, and the flow monitor is sounding an alarm. The sound is one that can't be ignored and quickly brings the nurse. She silences the alarm and removes the empty bag from its hook. Next, the Oxalipatin is connected via a Y-adapter to a larger bag of hydrating fluid before being routed through the monitor and programmed.

Having finished my ginger ale, I realize a bathroom break is needed. The device on the IV pole, however, is tethered to an electrical outlet. I ask the nurse how I might be set free for a few minutes, and she simply pulls the plug from the wall, assuring me the computer contains a battery that will take over temporarily. It feels somewhat naughty and daring to be walking away from the station that's been appointed Mother for the morning.

The recliners are filling up. Three nurses are kept busy setting up IV medication drips and responding to alarms from the monitoring devices. Some patients are cheerful and chatty, while others chose to read or watch television. Some slumber peacefully under warm blankets. I wonder why the majority of patients are female? The only man I see is in the station across from the bathroom. His companions are both wearing Corrections Canada uniforms.

The bathroom is roomier than most, so there's no lack of space for me and my tall friend with six feet who needs to be kept at arm's length so he doesn't trip me or step on my toes. I learn quickly that it's necessary to keep the pole moving as long as I'm moving. At first, I let go of the pole while facing the toilet, then turning to sit find myself wrapped in IV line. After reversing my turn, I grasp the pole, and *together* we assume the position. A large notice on the wall advises that chemotherapy patients are required to flush twice.

HESITANT HOPE

Back in my chair, I concentrate on the crossword puzzle and try to ignore the clear plastic line where a continuous stream of miniature warriors are marching into battle. Because the PICC line delivers them directly to my heart, they'll get a quick deployment to the front lines. Having finished his sudoku, and seeing I'm amused and comfortable, Sid wanders off to stretch his legs and find a coffee.

By the time the Oxalipatin pouch is empty, it's almost noon, and except for the tightness in my head and a strong desire to be cut loose, I have no other noticeable side effects.

The final steps involve the slow injection of a starter dose of Fluorouracil from a syringe and the attachment of the take-home bottle. For this procedure, my nurse dons a protective gown as well as rubber gloves. I'll carry the bottle in a black, zippered pouch held in place at my waist by an adjustable belt. The line exiting the bottle is fed upward beneath my shirt, then down the sleeve where it's connected to the PICC. The threaded, connecting components are screwed tightly together and taped for additional security. Wide gauze is wrapped around my arm numerous times to stabilize and protect the site, after which an elasticized mesh sleeve is added as the last protective layer.

The nurse gives me several plastic sleeves that I'll use to keep my arm dry when showering. At this point, another plastic bag arrives from the hospital pharmacy containing nausea medication to be taken at home. I also receive an orange package from the manufacturer of Oxalipatin containing thick rubberized gloves, a fleece face scarf, and reading material. Soon, I will notice a sensitivity to cold. I must wear the face scarf when going out and the gloves when taking containers from the refrigerator.

While waiting at the reception desk for appointment information, I reach for a sweet treat in the candy bowl. As I pop it into my mouth, the anticipation of the glorious butterscotch flavour is harshly intercepted by sharp pains in the muscles that are trying to close my jaws. My hands fly to my face. Slowly, the cramping passes and I am able to close my mouth. *What is that about?* I wonder.

With new appointment instructions tucked away, Sid helps me with my coat. In the hallway, a young lad of five or six with no hair pushes an IV pole along the hall outside the Children's Chemotherapy Unit, followed closely by his mother. I feel tears well. As we exit to the parking lot, I give thanks for sixty-three healthy years.

I'm fairly certain the belt, bottle, and IV line I'm wearing won't work with nightgowns, so we stop at the mall to purchase pyjamas—first a chemo shirt, now chemo PJs.

At home, I head to the refrigerator, but thoughts of lunch are momentarily side-tracked by the countdown sheet on the door.

"Exactly when is the appropriate time to allow myself the satisfaction of crossing off number 12? Should I wait until the infusion is complete on Thursday, or perhaps the end of the two-week cycle? No. I got up, I got dressed, and I showed up. This is the banner day! Where's my pencil?"

Thanks to the steroid medications that will help keep nausea at bay, sleep is out of the question. When it becomes obvious that fidgeting in bed is futile, I brew a cup of herbal tea then settle on the sofa with afghan, iPad, and the volumes of information provided by the medical community. I'm torn between the obligation I feel to continue educating myself about chemotherapy and the management of symptoms, and my desire to search the internet for every reference I can find to my disorder and the treatment available.

After wading further into the stack of chemo material, I continue my search at www.cancer.net, a website developed by the world's leading cancer doctors. There's a wealth of cancer-related information on this site, but my best effort fails to discover more than a brief reference to my diagnosis. What I'd really like to find is some prognostic data that would soothe my anxiety and provide assurance that the path I've chosen will lead to an outstanding result. Just tell me I'll be granted the privilege of waltzing merrily along for another ten to fifteen years. Is that too much to ask?

Weariness settles in—it's almost 2:30 a.m. I'll follow one last link then try again to get some sleep. The page that opens is a website called PMP Pals' Network. At Princess Margaret, my classification of treatment is called the Peritoneal Malignancy Program, but in this case, PMP stands for Pseudomyxoma Peritonei, an umbrella term under which fall the different types of appendix cancers as well as other peritoneal malignancies. Information on the homepage describes the website as a world-wide, volunteer, patient-advocacy program providing information and referrals as well as mentorship.

I feel a surge of excitement as testimonials from patients who've been treated for appendix cancer fill the screen. The testimonials laud the value of skilled physicians, proclaim treatment successes, and cheer survivals of ten-plus years. I soon realize, however, that each case is unique and may span an incredible array of variables.

With bated breath, I read a short paragraph on the prognosis for my malady:

"Many factors contribute to the prognosis of patients diagnosed with mucinous adenocarcinoma of the appendix. These factors may include pathology, staging, age and overall health, access to specialized care, etc."

Bated breath fizzles to a sigh as I set my research aside. After pouring a glass of water and turning out the lights, I shuffle to the bedroom. Why do I continue to look for answers I know can't be found?

While melting into pillow-soft comfort, my thoughts ricochet unabated. Wouldn't it be wonderful to share this journey with someone, a survivor, a mentor? Someone who's been through six months of chemotherapy, recovered from lengthy invasive surgery, and returned to an active lifestyle. I have solid support from Sid and my family, but none of them know what it feels like to stand in my shoes. I feel so alone.

Max nudges my hand and purrs softly as I stroke his head.

After a late breakfast, with pen and fresh notebook in hand, I begin charting my symptoms. There won't be much to say today, but as time passes my daily notes will become important guidelines for remaining treatments.

TREATMENT 1:

Day 1: Tue., Jan. 28/14. Temp. 36.6C (normal is 37.0C)
- *head began feeling tight during first hour of treatment*
- *jaw pain*
- *difficulty sleeping*

Day 2: Wed., Jan. 29/14. Temp. 35.9C
- *jaw pain*
- *sensitivity to cold on my hands and in my mouth*

I keep pulling the bottle out of its pouch to see if the contents are disappearing. At first, it's hard to tell, but by mid-morning on Wednesday the vacuum-sealed bag inside the bottle is noticeably flatter.

By the end of the second day, I need to use the insulated gloves. Touching a refrigerated container instantly creates the sensation of frostbite. I find it frustrating pulling the gloves on and off, but I'll adapt, won't I. The water pitcher, usually kept in the refrigerator, has a new home on the counter. Staying well hydrated is important considering the toxins that need to be flushed from my system once their work is done.

Day 3: Thur., Jan. 30/14. Temp. 36.5C. Infusion complete
- *feeling very unwell—fatigue and nausea*
- *noticing pain in thumb joint while I write*
- *head tight in temples and jaw*
- *need to sleep*

The nurse came today to remove the empty bottle. It felt so good to be rid of it. Not only was it an uncomfortable sleeping partner, but is undoubtedly to blame for how wretched I feel. I've been using the anti-nausea medication, but perhaps I need to increase the dosage.

The bristles on my toothbrush feel like wire.

Over the last four days, all the symptoms have done their level best to upstage one another:
- *fatigue and nausea*
- *heartburn and indigestion*
- *sore mouth—using baking soda rinse*
- *sensitivity to cold*
- *cramps, diarrhea, excessive gas*

If you think baked beans make you windy and malodorous, think again. Folfox beats the beans at least three times over. I frequently caution Sid to keep his distance, and there are times when he and Max simply leave the room.

By contrast, a sweet pleasure during this trial by chemicals is the vase of fresh cut flowers on the dining room table. For my birthday, Sandy arranged to have a bouquet delivered every two weeks. Even on the more difficult days, my spirits are lifted at the sight of such vibrant, natural beauty, particularly with snow swirling at the window. During my days of resurrection, I delight in clipping and rearranging the flowers when a change of water is needed. Sid smiles. He knows I'm back.

Days 8 and 9: Symptoms fading.

Day 10: Thur., Feb. 6/14. Temp. 36.4C
- *mouth better*
- *energy better*
- *no heartburn*
- *no diarrhea*

Days 11, 12, 13: No noticeable symptoms.

First cycle completed.
Tomorrow we begin again.
"Can I do this eleven more times? Just don't think about it. One day at a time."

The day prior to my second treatment finds me at the Cancer Centre with symptom journal in hand. After having blood drawn in the Chemo Unit, I complete the ESAS, then take a seat in the reception area to wait. It's a large room, and most of the seats are occupied.

"I wonder what my blood analysis will look like today? What will my body have to say about the toxic invasion? Will it work with me? Will it understand I'm doing what I think is best for both of us?"

When it's my turn, I take great pains to reveal every side effect experienced over the past two weeks. I don't want to leave anything out because I can't be sure what might be significant. Dr. Biagi listens carefully, asking questions to clarify each point. By the end of the interview, we are both satisfied that I am managing well. My blood-work results are available, and Dr. Biagi confirms I am ready for the next cycle at the same dosage.

My chemo shirt is fresh and clean, ready to fulfill its crucial role for the second time. I've summoned my brave face, but each step echoes dread.

Seated in the treatment recliner, I take care to ask the volunteer for ginger ale at room temperature. The treatment session goes without a hitch, but in short order my body begins to react with increasing displeasure. The jaw pain is now accompanied by a throbbing headache, and the fatigue—fatigue that no amount of rest alleviates—is back. When I step outside, the sensitivity to cold returns with a vengeance, the calves of my legs tingling as from a peppering of ice pellets. I press the fleece scarf to my nose and mouth, breathing as shallowly as I can. At home on the sofa, I massage both legs, hoping to relieve the ache in once-strong quadriceps. Max is at my side extending a paw, pressing his soft warm pads into my arm. With eyes riveted to mine, I acknowledge his concern, certain of his desire to comfort.

My hands and feet tingle, not as when exposed to cold, but rather like they've fallen asleep. I want to cry, "What's happening to me?" But I *know* what's happening to me. I've been told, and I've read. I know I'm experiencing what's considered normal for a chemotherapy patient on Folfox, but I feel abused, tortured. I'm being poisoned.

I've agreed to this. I've given my consent.

It hurts anyway.

TREATMENT 2:

Day 1: Tue., Feb. 11/14. Temp. 38.2C
- *nausea and fatigue (one nausea pill)*
- *legs ache*
- *jaw pain and headache*
- *cold sensitivity*
- *numbness and tingling in hands, feet, and calves*
- *fever with red blotches on face and chest*

By evening, my temperature rises to 38.2C where it remains for over an hour, triggering a trip to the Emergency with my fever card. The waiting area is a zoo. It will be a while before I can expect to be triaged, and I'm already worried about what my compromised immune system is being exposed to. Masks are available, so I slip one on while we wait. Finally summoned, I explain my situation to the nurse. She immediately slides a thermometer into my mouth, 37.6C. This creates a dilemma. I'm no longer in the danger zone. The triage nurse is willing to process me, but because no beds are available Sid and I decide to go home and continue monitoring my temperature. We know a return trip will take only minutes.

The night ends well.

Day 2: Wed., Feb. 12/14. Temp. 37.6C
- *nausea and fatigue (two nausea pills)*
- *jaw pain and headache (acetaminophen)*
- *flushing in face, neck, and chest*
- *cold sensitivity*
- *numbness and tingling in hands, feet, and calves*
- *flavour of food changes*

I have a metallic taste in my mouth. The tuna fish in my sandwich doesn't taste like tuna fish. The taste of anything from a metal container seems distorted. Sid will have to choose glass, plastic or tetra packs when he shops.

Day 3: Thur., Feb. 13/14. Temp. 36.8C. Infusion complete
- *nausea and fatigue (two nausea pills)*
- *flushing*
- *jaw pain*
- *heartburn and indigestion*
- *mouth sore, tongue swollen (mouthwash 3 times)*
- *cold sensitivity*
- *numbness and tingling in fingers intensifies*

When the empty bottle is removed, I once again descend into a nauseous stupor and collapse in my bed where I'll sleep for the next twenty-four hours, waking only for drinks and bathroom breaks. Sid is usually close by when I awake, sometimes kneeling at the side of the bed, watching me, feeling helpless. For several days of each cycle, he shops, prepares meals, and does the laundry while I'm too ill to take any interest in the daily routine. When he quizzes me about what I feel like eating, I ask for soup, pudding, or a smoothie.

Day 4: Fri., Feb. 14/14. Temp. 36.9C
- *nausea and fatigue (two nausea pills)*
- *heartburn and indigestion*
- *cold sensitivity*
- *jaw and thumb pain*
- *tongue swollen and sore (mouthwash 3 times)*
- *numbness in fingers*

It's Valentine's Day. Rather unlike any Valentine's Day I can recall. The romance associated with the event seems remote. There are no preparations for a candle-lit dinner for two in an upscale restaurant, no wine, and no chocolates. Instead, quiet, steady devotion flowing from the strong to the weak, "in sickness and in health, till death do us part."

Day 5: Sat., Feb. 15/14. Temp. 36.8C
- *jaw pain less intense*
- *nausea and fatigue (one nausea pill)*
- *cold sensitivity fading*
- *numbness and tingling in hands fading*
- *mouth and tongue improving*

After soaking my toothbrush in a glass of warm water, I gingerly touch it to my teeth trying to stay clear of the gums and tongue. This is not good. Oral hygiene at its worst.

HESITANT HOPE

Day 6: Sun., Feb. 16/14. Temp. 36.8C
- *still some jaw pain*
- *fatigue*
- *mouth still tender*
- *cramping, diarrhea*

The bathroom is very popular with me these days. A sudoku book helps pass the time. Think I'll ask for a padded seat.

Days 7 and 8: Temp. 37.0C
- *fatigue less severe*
- *mouth improving*
- *heartburn improves with medication*
- *cramping, diarrhea*

The fatigue is finally fading. I'd like to get outside for a short walk and some fresh air, maybe accompany Sid to the grocery store. I could push the cart. There's a bathroom.

Days 9 through 12:
- *energy improves*
- *appetite improves, but not the taste*
- *nose very dry*
- *hair begins to thin*

I'm disappointed to see an unusually large number of hairs around my feet in the shower. Wiping the steam from the bathroom mirror, I run a comb through my hair. Will there be enough to get me through five more months. I wipe a tear from my cheek and blow my nose. There's blood on the tissue.

6
ONE DAY AT A TIME

*Yea, though I walk through the valley
of the shadow of death ...*

—Psalm 23:4

My life must be more than a symptom journal if I'm to make it through a total of twelve treatments with my sanity intact. I need to get a life beyond chemotherapy.

Experience has taught me that days nine through fourteen are when I should schedule activities and outings that will add much needed zest to an otherwise depressing routine. Even days one and two are options because I'm reasonably well until all the drugs are on board.

My Christmas gift certificates are waiting on the clock shelf and spur me to make a search of the internet, for once unrelated to my medical concern. On the Grand Theatre website, a Bruce Cockburn concert captures my interest, and after confirming that Adam is free on February 22, I book two tickets. Not only do I look forward to being entertained by one of the artists whose music was part of my early years, but also to spending an intimate evening with my son, whose schedule is very demanding.

Helen DeVries

And the cat's in the cradle and the silver spoon
Little boy blue and the man in the moon.[1]

Unlike Valentine's Day which fell on day four—positively the worst day of the two-week cycle—dinner and a concert are possible on day eleven. My energy level is far from ideal, but an afternoon nap will hopefully provide the stamina I need.

After choosing two favourite pieces from my closet, black wool dress pants to be worn over warm tights, and a glitzy red top, I search my jewelry box for the perfect earrings. I lean toward the mirror expecting my fingers to perform their nimble magic. They can't identify the edges of the small clasp. I look down. My thumb and index finger are in position, but they are not sensing the tiny circular piece of metal between them. I pinch my digits together tightly and continue, trying to align the clasp with the end of the post piercing my earlobe. They fail to connect. Looking at my hand again, I see the clasp has turned sideways in my grip. With both hands working together, I reposition the clasp and try again ... and again ... and again. Beads of perspiration form on my forehead, cheekbones, and upper lip. How frustrating. I could ask for help, but I fear Sid's larger hands would serve him no better than my numb pegs. I need to sit for a moment. At last, I realize a pair of one-piece earrings will solve my dilemma.

Sid is preparing dinner as Adam and I leave. The sweet anticipation of this coveted evening cannot preclude pangs of guilt as I leave my faithful caregiver behind to prepare yet another meal while I prepare to paint the town.

Adam and I walk hand in hand from the parking garage, the snow crunching underfoot, our breath forming small white

---

1   Harry Chapin

clouds that scurry over our shoulders at the same hurried pace of passersby. I'll savour each moment, committing all to memory like funds to a savings account—the eye-catching displays in shop windows, the sweet smell of gourmet offerings on our table, the nurture of relaxed conversation, the bliss of treasured melodies, the satisfaction of time well spent.

The day before my third treatment, I have the usual lab work prior to meeting with my oncologist. I learn a CEA test has been done to measure tumour markers in my blood. The result shows a significant reduction of these markers when compared to the same test done before treatment began. This is a good indicator the Folfox therapy is having the desired effect.

The bloody nose that's been a concern for several days is nothing to worry about I'm told. The chemotherapy is drying my tissues, but this problem can be managed by regular lubrication with an over-the-counter nasal gel.

For the irritation in my mouth, Dr. Biagi prescribes Magic Mouthwash, a pleasant tasting antibiotic, anti-fungal, and corticosteroid liquid, to be used several times a day for a two-minute rinse, then swallowed for the benefit of the esophagus and stomach.

The fever and rash that accompanied treatment two are of concern, prompting a change in the infusion rate of Oxalipatin from two to three hours.

I'm cleared for treatment three.

Earlier in the month, I declined an invitation to attend a Look Good Feel Good workshop at the Cancer Centre, but now I'm ready to see if the next opportunity falls on one of my better days. March 12, day two of treatment four, should work, and while we're thinking about looking good, let's make an appointment to get my hair done.

TREATMENT 3: *February 25, 2014*

In spite of the slower infusion rate for the Oxalipatin, I run a fever of 37.6C with some rashing on the second day. My nose is extremely dry because new symptoms of sneezing and congestion have increased my need to blow. I'm thankful for the nasal gel and apply it frequently. The joint pain that was initially only in my thumbs is now in my knees and hips. Through the difficult days of this treatment, my sights are set on day twelve when we'll travel to Ottawa to celebrate Adam's fortieth birthday with family and friends at the Mill Street Brew Pub on the Ottawa River. It's precisely occasions like this that pull me—like metal to a magnet—when considering the reasons to accept treatment and go on living.

"Just who do I think I'm fooling with this *looking ahead to happy times* charade? It does nothing to alter the reality of where I'm headed. Face it, Kiddo, that pathetic little light at the end of the tunnel could flicker and die at any moment. One bad CT scan and you're toast."

The clouds have gathered again. Darkness. Grief. Hopelessness.

The view from the living room window is as bleak as my mood. I stare at the fragmented ice floes lying helpless in the black, frigid water of the bay twelve stories below. They have no means of escape. Iron-clad docking walls, a steep and rocky shoreline, and a prevailing westerly wind hold them captive. Victims of circumstance.

HESITANT HOPE

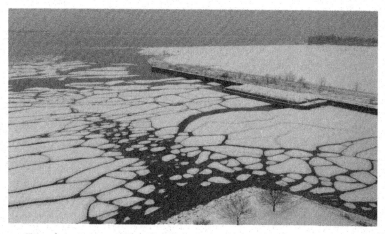

For the past month, I've been weighing the pros and cons of seeking a mentor through the online PMP Pals' Network. The first step is to register and pay a membership fee, but for some reason I can't bring myself to do it. Am I being too cautious? Surely the organization would make every effort to ensure my mentor is a good match. If the match is less than ideal, how would I know? I'm afraid of being drawn off-track. I want this relationship, but I'm not willing to accept the risk. I have enough uncertainty to deal with at the moment. I will try to be satisfied with the trust I have in my doctors and the support of my family.

During the best days of cycle three, I'm blessed with numerous visits from friends and relatives. Each provides support in their own unique way, and I strive to be open and accepting to every offering whether it be hugs, words of encouragement, pleasant conversation, or a sympathetic glance. I know each of them, regardless of their faith or lack thereof, is praying in their own way for my recovery. These wonderful people don't realize how much their gestures mean.

TREATMENT 4: *March 11, 2014*

The Look Good Feel Good event on March 12, twenty-four hours before the fourth infusion is complete, is a very uplifting experience. The seminar is attended by ten ladies, and the first order of business is to present each with a generous make-up kit to compliment her complexion. An experienced make-up artist demonstrates the proper use of the products and provides hands-on assistance. Information about wigs is also given with the opportunity to try different colours and styles. In my case, a wig shouldn't be necessary, but for many chemotherapy patients it will make a huge difference in how they feel about themselves. I return home feeling better and looking great. Too bad it won't last.

My body is showing less resilience—a wounded warrior.

Mild fevers come and go, my sensitivity to cold worsens, and the weakness is more pronounced with dizzy spells and trembling thrown in. My need for sleep has increased, which means less physical activity, which leads to even more weakness—a vicious circle. The numbness and tingling in my hands and feet are becoming problematic. My fingertips are smooth and slippery with no evidence of fingerprints, causing me to fumble and drop objects frequently. The palms of my hands and the soles of my feet appear to have a mild sunburn.

At the next pre-treatment interview, Dr. Biagi listens attentively to my concerns. After a few questions, a decision is made to decrease the dosage of Oxalipatin by ten percent, a reduction not considered significant enough to compromise the effectiveness of the treatment, but hopefully enough to dampen the more troublesome symptoms.

HESITANT HOPE

TREATMENT 5: *March 25, 2014*

There's the bell. It's round five. Remember the confidence and determination I felt stepping into the ring for round one? I'm a fighter. I can do this. But with each round, I've been bruised and bloodied. I retreat to my corner after each assault for a period of relief and the encouragement of my coaches, but I'm no match for this opponent. I want the bell to ring for the last time. I want this to be over.

As soon as the lengthy infusion in the Chemotherapy Unit is complete, I notice the jaw pain is significantly reduced. The other symptoms, however, return as usual with the sensitivity to cold in my fingers being more severe.

I've been trying to ignore indications that my brain is being affected by the chemical cocktails, but it's no use. The unwelcome forgetfulness I've thus far attributed to aging and the hormonal changes of menopause has been frustratingly magnified. The overabundance of eggs in the refrigerator is only one of the embarrassing reminders.

"We need eggs," I stated while pushing the grocery cart yesterday.

"I think we bought eggs on the last trip," Sid suggests.

"No. I'm sure we need eggs."

I've been getting angry with Sid for interrupting me when I'm relating events. Why does he suddenly think his recall is so much better than mine? I've always been good with details, or I *was* until now. Honestly, I'm not sure of anything anymore.

Conversation is frustrating. In the amount of time it takes for me to formulate my thoughts for a comment, the subject has changed. My speech is slower, and often a word will refuse to come leaving me silent mid-sentence. For one who's never been at a loss for words and enjoys a spirited discussion, finding myself in this state of mental deterioration is unbearable.

Focus is also an issue. It's not unusual for me to read the same paragraph a second or third time before I feel I've grasped the content fully. I looked forward to reading as a pleasant way to while away the hours of illness, but mastering a book has become an arduous task.

We're talking about quality of life issues. Will these side effects completely recede when this is over, or will I be left with distressing reminders of my decision to pursue treatment? How much am I sacrificing for this attempt at a longer lifespan? How much am I *willing* to sacrifice? Just how does one measure quality of life? Certainly, it's more than just being here, more than simply drawing breath.

Once again, a bit of advanced planning is the broom that sweeps the sobering thoughts from my mind. In a few minutes, my favourite ladies will pick me up for a lunch date. When I look at my daughter and granddaughter, two generations carrying unmistakable familial characteristics, I feel strengthened. I'm part of an ancestral chain with vibrant links reaching into the future. This is a concept I no longer take for granted.

In November, when it was determined the cancer originated in my appendix rather than my ovary, Dr. Martin had been quick to reassure me that for Sandy and Hailey this was a very positive finding because ovarian cancer has such a strong hereditary link. Appendix cancer, it's believed, doesn't share this link. I can only pray it's so.

TREATMENT 6: April 8, 2014

This treatment puts me at the halfway point. There is some satisfaction in reaching this median marker, but mostly I dread what's still to come. A CT scan has been ordered for April 16, and I'm hopeful the results will fall in line with those of the tumour marker test giving me the encouragement I need to face the final six.

Sid and I will celebrate our forty-sixth wedding anniversary on April 20. That's a lot of years filled with memories—many happy, some not. We're not strangers to adversity, but this year trumps them all, leaving us to wonder how many anniversaries remain. Whenever possible, I choose not to think about the future—unless I feel the need for a good cry.

Our children and grandchildren have gathered for this special day. *They* obviously wish to think about the future—a future with me in it. Their gift to us is a custom-made wooden sign with our first names carved above a painting of two graceful swans on a peaceful lake bathed in evening sun, our surname painted boldly across the bottom. We'll find the perfect place to display this beautiful tribute at our RV this summer.

After I visit the lab and chat with Lou, Sid and I wait nervously for the doctor to appear on April 22. We take turns pacing and gazing out the window with feigned interest. There's usually a bit of a wait because the results of the lab work are needed for a complete assessment.

Dr. Dancey is working in the clinic today and arrives with a smile and handshake. She conducts a short physical exam, checking the lymph nodes for swelling and the abdomen for changes. Her advice for the red, cracked skin on my feet is to moisturize frequently with an alcohol-free cream.

"You want to hear about your CT scan," she says, opening the file and perusing the report. "It shows a slight reduction of the cancer tissue."

A sigh of relief escapes my lips as they form a hopeful smile.

"This is a positive result, but we need to wait and see what the next scan shows. This doesn't necessarily mean surgery will be possible."

Another reality check.

"I understand."

TREATMENT 7: April 23, 2014

The dark days of this cycle pass in the usual way—aching muscles and joints, nausea, diarrhea, extreme drowsiness and weakness, cold sensitivity, numbness and cracked skin on my hands and feet, and an inflamed mouth.

When my worst days have passed, Betty Ann visits again bringing more home-cooked foods she hopes I'll enjoy. Over the weekend, we're thrilled to welcome visitors John and Sharon from New Brunswick and Marion from Ancaster.

Marion lost her husband, George, to cancer at the age of fifty. I still remember the day they broke the news of his illness. We were enjoying cocktails before dinner at our home, the four of us in our mid-to-late forties, healthy and living the good life. Sid and George took the occasional fishing trip together, and as couples we enjoyed several boating vacations on the Rideau Canal, St. Lawrence River and Lake Ontario.

The news was shocking. Lung cancer. We offered our sympathy, but once those two words were uttered the atmosphere changed from relaxed and cheerful to tense and somber. An elephant was sucking the air out of the room.

It pains me to say we travelled to Ancaster only once during George's lengthy decline. Considering the happy times shared over the years, we failed miserably to provide the support due such a friendship. Now, the shoe is on the other foot. Not only do we understand how difficult it is to set one's inhibitions aside and commit to spending time with a family member or friend who is gravely ill, we also know how important small amounts of time are when given consistently over the period of illness.

TREATMENT 8: *May 6, 2014*

Yesterday, I was cleared for another treatment. Dr. Biagi didn't say the problem with my feet wasn't serious. What he *did* say was that he has patients whose symptoms make them feel like they're walking over hot coals. Translation? I should thank my lucky stars.

The excitement for my better days of this cycle involves the delivery of our RV to the campground in Adolphustown. After being in storage over the winter, it resumes the roll of summer cottage. The camping season always begins with a Saturday morning devoted to clearing the branches left behind by winter winds and ice, followed by a barbecue. Unfortunately, the weather forecast is cold and windy for Saturday, so I'll delay my first visit until the setup is complete and I can be warm and comfortable. I hope the change of scenery will be refreshing, and activities such as Friday afternoon card games will make the time seem to pass more quickly so I can get to the end of these dreadful treatments.

TREATMENT 9: *May 21, 2014*

Spring is definitely in the air. I've tucked a scarf into my bag, but I'm hoping to breathe deeply of the fresh, mild air without the need to protect my cold-sensitive airway. Few seats remain in the reception area when we arrive at the Chemotherapy Unit. Once settled, I notice a lady who reminds me of someone I knew years ago. I turn to Sid and ask if she looks familiar. When I look back in her direction, she's coming toward us.

"Are you Sid DeVries?"

"I am. Helen was just saying she thought we should know you."

Over thirty years ago, we attended the same church as Corry when we lived in Kingston the first time. Our daughters were friends, but contact was lost after we moved to Ottawa.

"It's so nice to see you again, but the fact that we're meeting here can't be a good thing. Which one of you is receiving treatment?" Corry inquires.

After a brief summary of my situation, I learn she's being treated for ovarian cancer. Corry acknowledges her treatment is palliative, but is feeling quite well and making the most of her time.

"This didn't need to happen," she explains with regret. "When I had a hysterectomy several years ago, I asked the doctor to take my ovaries as well, but following the surgery I was told my ovaries were healthy and didn't need to be removed. So here I am. But what's worse," she continues sadly, "my son-in-law is also being treated here for colon cancer. He's in his early forties."

Our conversation is interrupted by a nurse announcing Corry's name.

"See you inside," she says as she turns away.

"Wasn't that a lovely surprise to see Corry again after so many years?" I say, turning to Sid. "But such heartbreaking circumstances."

"Helen DeVries."

That's my cue.

The process has become second nature. The nursing staff, who do their jobs so well, are like family. When I unplug midway through my infusion for a trip to the bathroom, I'm surprised to see another familiar face. Stuart was another member of the same congregation from thirty-plus years ago. What an unusual coincidence. Stuart's story is also very sad. He has esophageal cancer and is receiving his first treatment today. As with Corry, there is no hope for a cure. He's been given less than three years.

I'm feeling fortunate. How strange is that? I have a precious commodity my friends do not—a small grain of hope.

TREATMENT 10: June 3, 2014

Double digits! It feels like I'm nearing the end. Only two more after this one. One more month. Sid's been afraid that at some point I'd become reluctant to continue, simply refusing to get out of bed on treatment morning. That I willingly accept infusion after infusion knowing what the following week brings has him in awe of my stamina and determination.

Sid worries about me, and I worry about him. What toll has the stress and added responsibilities of the last seven months taken? He isn't one to let his feelings show, nor does he care to talk about them. His attitude is, "It is what it is. Deal with it." Nevertheless, I encourage him to return to some of the activities he was involved in before I became ill. Since October, he's ignored his part-time employment as an Inspector for the Chief Firearms Office, but if I arrange to have a friend in for the day and tell him there's no need for him to be here, maybe he'll decide to schedule a work day, or, better yet, a golf day with the guys. Our time at the RV works well because he can be outside chatting with other campers while still close enough to keep tabs on me. I'm thankful we're dealing with this in our retirement when our time is our own. That factor alone puts us miles ahead—no jobs, no children at home, just the two of us.

Friends Grant and Donna join us for an entertaining afternoon of *Driving Miss Daisy* at the Thousand Islands Playhouse in Gananoque on June 13. Two days later, we enjoy dinner with

Sandy and Geoff at their home in Roblin. One more day until it begins again.

TREATMENT 11: June 17, 2014

The numbness in my fingers is seriously affecting my ability to perform basic tasks like buttoning my blouse, so my dosage has been reduced by another ten percent. I'm concerned about what these reductions mean in terms of the effectiveness of the treatments, but I understand we're trying to maintain a fine balance between therapeutic benefit and quality of life.

Another family celebration for Hailey's nineteenth birthday takes place on June 29, two days before my final treatment. I'm so fortunate all of our special occasions have taken place during the second week of my cycles.

TREATMENT 12: July 2, 2014

Lou was right. This is a difficult day. I thought I'd be happy knowing this is the last one, but I'm bone-tired, too drained to feel happiness. Hopefully, when the worst days of this final assault are over, I'll be pleasantly surprised by the return of positive feelings.

"This is my last treatment," I tell the nurse, once settled in the treatment recliner.

"Are you sure?" she responds.

How could I *not* be sure? I can't believe she's asking me this.

"Yes, twelve cycles was the deal, and this is the twelfth."

When you walk through the doors of the Chemotherapy Unit, one of the first things you notice to your left is a shiny brass bell anchored to the wall. I have passed that bell on twelve occasions. My treatment schedule is complete. I have earned the right!

CLANG, CLANG! CLANG, CLANG! CLANG, CLANG!

7

MAKING THE CUT

There is no hope unmingled with fear,
and no fear unmingled with hope.

—Baruch Spinoza

"Take a breath and hold it," the giant doughnut instructs. I lie inside his immenseness while he evaluates with whirring and clicking.

"Breathe."

His long, soft tongue, on which I've been positioned with my arms above my head, delivers me back to the technician.

"I'm going to inject the dye now, Mrs. DeVries," the technician advises, "and remember, it will make you feel like you've wet yourself—a sensation only. Are you ready?"

"I am."

No, not really. The infusion from my final treatment isn't yet complete, I've sipped my way through the unpleasant pre-CT aperitif, and I'm being injected with dye, not to mention the radiation from Mr. Doughnut.

Ah, there's that nice warm feeling I've come to expect.

I'm being swallowed up again.

"Take a breath and hold it."

The scan is extensive—only my head, arms and legs are excluded. "Breathe."

With the imaging complete, the technician removes the IV catheter used to inject the dye and helps me to a sitting position.

"That's it, Mrs. DeVries, we're finished. We'd like you to sit in the waiting area for fifteen minutes so we can be sure there'll be no allergic reaction, then you can be on your way."

The conflict between the need to know and the fear of knowing are constantly in play, pushing and pulling, retreating and advancing in my brain. My next appointment with Dr. Biagi is ten days away—ten days that will be spent worrying while trying not to worry.

Over the last eight months, I've tried to understand the differing mindsets of people who know they have a life-threatening illness and those who are confident in their state of wellness. Those in my group experience significant fear and anxiety, while most in the second group go matter-of-factly about their daily routine with little concern for tomorrow, in spite of the fact that all of us know death is inevitable and can come at any time.

The second group is like a man walking a subway line, earbuds in place, unaware a train is bearing down on him from behind. The first group is like a man walking the subway line who sees the train approaching, but has no means of escape.

I see the train.

At home, I no more than hang my coat in the closet before the nurse arrives to remove the last spent chemo bottle. The PICC site has become a problem over the past several weeks. The skin on the inside of my upper arm is badly irritated from dressing after dressing held in place by adhesives that my skin will no longer tolerate. I've asked the nurse to use a gauze wrap rather than adhesive to give the skin a chance to heal.

"Will you be removing the PICC line today?" I ask expectantly.

After checking her paperwork, she replies, "No, I don't have a requisition to remove it."

Disappointment washes over me. I know the intruder has saved me much poking and jabbing with needles and has been an excellent delivery system for the drugs, but I'm *so* ready to be rid of it. I'd love to shower *sans* plastic sleeve and choose blouses without considering the sleeve length. My next opportunity won't be until July 14, when I return to the clinic for follow-up. Oh well. For the next five days, I'll be too miserable to care, then Adam, Samuel, and William will be visiting for a few days so time will pass quickly.

The weekend is a blur of nausea and exhaustion, but it's finally starting to sink in—*this is the last time!* No more agonizing rehearsals on treatment mornings, and no more painful days of recovery. I'm sure it will take a while to get my strength back, but at least the clubbing has stopped. When this all began in January, I couldn't even conceive of being where I am today—*at the end*. I really did make it!

Sid gets me settled at the RV before Adam and the boys arrive. Normally, we'd have our grandsons for several days on our own, but this year Adam will be chief caregiver for their three-day stay.

"Watch me ride my bike, Grandma!"

"Grandma, can we have a popsicle?"

"Grandma, can you come to the beach with us?"

It feels great to be in demand. I manage the short walk to the beach, and once in my lawn chair under shady branches, I'm entertained by Sam and Will for hours as they construct a village with sand and bucket after bucket of water from the shoreline.

"Grandma, come look at the road I built."

"That's a great road, Sam!"

"Look at my castle, Grandma."

"Amazing, William! I think I'd like to live in *this* village."

When it's time for parting hugs and kisses, my heart is full. What a wonderful few days this has been. These are the days I don't want to miss.

In spite of my status as an observer, I'm exhausted. The walks to the beach and the playground have sapped my energy, and my desire not to miss anything saw me up and about when I probably should have been lying down. I know my strength will gradually return, but that too, will require determination.

Finally, it's Monday, July 14, appointment day. I'm to have the usual lab work done at 8:15 a.m. before seeing Dr. Biagi. I think nothing of the requested lab evaluation until my pre-appointment talk with Lou.

"It feels so good to know there will be no treatment tomorrow," I bubble, as I take a seat in the examining room.

"What do you mean?" Lou asks in a serious tone.

"I mean I'm finished. I've had twelve treatments."

"Are you sure?"

I can't believe this! I deserve a hug, or at the very least a congratulatory handshake, but it's just another day of seeing one cancer patient after another. I understand that remembering every detail in every file is impossible, but a simple acknowledgement of what I've accomplished, what I've endured, would mean a lot.

"I want to get my PICC line removed."

"I'll mention that to Dr. Biagi. He'll see you shortly."

My intention to wait calmly is short-lived. Repeated crossing and uncrossing of legs along with thumb-twiddling signals my fading repose. It's time to check out this small space: an examination table covered with a fresh sheet of paper; a counter with sink; a dispenser of paper cups; cupboards, above and below; boxes of latex gloves in small, medium, and large; instructions on how to wash your hands; a rack of symptom evaluation forms—I wonder if it's for people who fail to complete the computerized version, or whether it's merely a has-been awaiting permanent removal. There's also a note taped to a cupboard door that instructs regarding the scheduling of appointments, but the procedure described doesn't seem to fall in line with what I've experienced. I wonder what's going on in the hall?

Dr. Biagi seldom travels without a resident in tow, and on many occasions the student carries out a preliminary evaluation before he enters the exam room. I'd prefer bypassing the extra questions and just get to the scan results.

When all the questions have been answered and the examining is finished, Dr. Biagi picks up my file.

"I have the results of your last scan, Mrs. DeVries, and it shows no change from the scan we did three months ago."

I'm dumbfounded. No change? How is that possible? How could three more months, six more treatments not make a difference?

"I've been in touch with your Toronto team and brought them up-to-date on your progress. Dr. McCart would like to see you there on Friday."

"Friday? She wants to see me this Friday?" This is as shocking as the scan report.

"Yes, she'll see you at 11:40 a.m. on Friday to review your scans and discuss the possibility of surgery. I understand you'd like to have your PICC line removed."

"Yes, please." Finally, something I understand.

"Stop at the Chemotherapy Unit before you leave and one of the nurses there will take care of that for you. We also need to schedule an appointment for you to see me again in two weeks."

I'm devastated by the scan results. Please don't tell me I endured twelve chemotherapy treatments for nothing. I'm surprised Dr. McCart even wants to see me. I'm sure it will be to tell me I don't qualify for her surgery.

For the last six months, I've concentrated on putting one foot in front of the other, getting from one treatment to the next, so much so that the bigger picture blurred. It's time to lift my head, adjust my focus, reaffirm the knowledge that chemotherapy was merely a prerequisite—a first step. Will it also be the last?

The obstacles standing between me and a brighter future are clear once again.

The trip to Toronto begins early Friday morning with a brief stop in Napanee to collect Sandy, who is taking the day off to join us. After an initial burst of conversation, we fall silent. Reclining my seat slightly, I turn my head and gaze at the puffy, white clouds floating in a bright, blue sky. I search for whimsical profiles as the wind licks their edges. This is therapy—cloud therapy—used since childhood as a distraction from life's harsher moments. The little light at the end of the tunnel is flickering precariously.

We arrive at Princess Margaret Hospital with plenty of time to spare. It's easier this time, less stressful. We know where to park, which entrance to use, and where to find the elevators and the Gastrointestinal Clinic. After checking in at reception, we select seats and make ourselves comfortable. The waiting area has at least fifty chairs, most of them occupied. Assuming every patient brought at least one family member, the actual number of people with appointments is likely less than half. Perhaps we should have grabbed an early lunch in the deli on the first floor.

"I think I'll go downstairs and pick up a few snacks, Mom. Anything in particular you fancy?" Sandy was reading my thoughts.

HESITANT HOPE

It's shortly after 1 p.m. when Dr. McCart enters the examination room where we've waited for some time, in addition to the hour in reception.

After I introduce Sandy, Dr. McCart begins.

"I understand you've completed twelve cycles of Folfox."

"Yes. The last treatment was on July 2."

"Did you have any problems?"

"I did. It was necessary to reduce the Oxalipatin because of numbness in my hands and feet. I worried the treatments would be less effective, but I also understood why it was necessary."

"You appear to be doing well. Can I check your abdomen?"

"Certainly," I respond, positioning myself on the examination table. "I *am* doing well, but I'm still very tired and weak."

Dr. McCart nods. "We've had a good look at your scans. The one done partway through your treatments shows a small reduction of the tumour tissue in your abdomen. The last one shows no change."

"No change after the last six cycles can't be a good thing," I add in a regretful tone.

"I'm not too concerned about that," replies Dr. McCart.

This is *not* what I was expecting to hear. Since my appointment on Monday, I've been living in fear that there is nowhere left for me to go in terms of viable treatment. What a roller-coaster ride! Fear ... Hope ... Despair ... Hope ...

"What's more important," Dr. McCart continues, "is that we don't see anything outside of your abdomen. That's a good thing, a very good thing. What I'd like to do next is schedule you for a laparoscopy. We would admit you and do it in the OR under anesthetic. It involves making an incision so we can insert a small camera and have a good look around to see just how much tumour tissue there is in your abdomen and where it's located. If we think we can remove all of it, then we would schedule you for the big operation, the one that could take up to twenty hours.

"In order for you to benefit from this surgery, we must be able to remove all visible signs of cancer, then the HIPEC treatment would take care of the remaining microscopic cells. The other very important consideration is that the cancer must not be attached to any organs you can't live without—your small intestines, for example."

"So at this point, you still don't know whether I will be scheduled for surgery?"

"Correct."

"But you will know after you complete the laparoscopy?"

"Yes. Do you have any other questions?"

"I've read your patient education booklet several times, so I understand everything you've said. The questions that remain are questions you don't have answers for yet."

"Do you wish me to schedule the laparoscopy?" Dr. McCart asks.

"Yes, if you still think I'm a good candidate for your surgery, I would like to continue."

"Very well. The next opportunity is on July 31. We'll admit you the day before so we can do some tests and prepare you for the procedure. You'll be in the OR for about one hour. The procedure involves making a small incision below the navel so we can insert a tube that will be used to introduce some gas into your abdomen. This will make it easier for us to move about once we insert the miniature camera that will let us examine the surfaces of the abdominal organs as well as the peritoneal lining. Depending on how well you recover after the anesthetic wears off, we may release you the same day, but you should plan to stay in Toronto overnight as a precaution."

As in December when Dr. McCart first explained the possibility of a life-saving option, my mind races the entire trip home. Once again, I've grabbed a merciful branch on the slippery slope that ends in the valley of terminal disease.

HESITANT HOPE

Patients selected as candidates for this surgery must meet the following criteria:

- Less than 70 years of age
- BMI < 35
- In good general health
- No extra-peritoneal disease
- No tumours on vital organs
- Surgeon must feel that all visible disease can be removed

I now qualify under four of six criteria.

It's less than two weeks until the next procedure—less than two weeks for me to cycle through the next vortex of emotion. I rejoice in clearing one more hurdle. I cheer at the sight of my little candle of hope burning with a renewed glow of possibility. But slowly, unwillingly, I'm consumed by the insatiable fear of rejection. Will I meet the demands of the remaining criteria? Is the branch I'm clinging to strong enough, or will I be sucked into the dark, angry mudslide of despair?

As fate would have it, I develop an upper respiratory infection a few days after my Toronto visit. At a follow-up appointment in Kingston with Dr. Dancey on July 28, a chest x-ray is ordered to rule out pneumonia. I place a call to Dr. McCart and reluctantly explain my situation. Will she allow the exploratory laparoscopy to proceed or will she postpone? She feels that because I no longer have a fever and am improving, there is very little risk.

On Wednesday, July 30, we travel to Toronto again. This time we navigate the admission process at Mount Sinai Hospital. Once settled in my room, preparations begin for the laparoscopic procedure that will take place in the morning. The afternoon flies by as an IV catheter is installed, blood samples taken, ECG performed, medical history reviewed, and an anesthetist and respiratory therapist question me. I relate the details of my recent cold symptoms to each specialist to ensure they have no concerns. It bothers me that the patient in the next bed, as well as her mother, can hear every word.

While I'm occupied with medical staff, Sid checks in at the nearby Eaton Chelsea Hotel where he's pleased to be offered a compassionate rate for a hospital-related stay. I'm looking forward to joining him there tomorrow provided all goes well. In the late afternoon, he returns to keep me company. The view of a bustling city from my window on the fourteenth floor preempts conversation, as together we watch the shadows lengthen and nightfall overtake the city.

"I'll be back first thing tomorrow before they take you to the OR," he whispers after a long embrace.

The busy daytime pace of hospital life has slowed. Visitors are saying their goodbyes. The mother of the young lady in the next bed is fussing about, making sure her daughter's every need is met before she leaves. The view from the window is now about lights—lights from buildings, lights from street lamps, lights from moving vehicles, and lights from billboards. The city is so big, this hospital is big, my problem is big—all looming over me like the menacing shadows of ghouls and goblins at Halloween. I feel small and alone.

I don't know what to think, what to feel. I have to decide, take control. I can feel fear—fear that the result of tomorrow's procedure won't be favourable and I'll be dismissed from the Peritoneal Malignancy Program. I can feel thankful—thankful that I'm living in this decade when medical science believes they have a solution to my problem. I can feel confident—confident that the result of the exploratory will be good, putting me one step closer to the possibility of a cure. I'll sleep better if I choose the latter.

HESITANT HOPE

Before I know it, Sid is there holding my hand as I'm swept off to surgery.

"I'll be waiting," I hear him say as his hand slips from mine.

I can't remember waking up in Recovery, but Sid says we chatted a bit. My first recollection is of entering a room with two freshly made beds. Why am I not being returned to the room I left this morning? The nurses deliver me to the bed near the window, then busy themselves removing the unoccupied furnishings. I have no objection to a private room, but I'm a little confused by the unusual activity.

Soon, a nurse arrives carrying a lab kit.

"We need to check you for infection," she says, removing a swab-shaped brush from sterile packaging. "I need to collect some nasal tissue with this brush, and it's going to hurt. I have to insert it firmly as far as it will go so the end will bend and follow the curve into the nasal cavity."

Ouch! She's right. Nothing like a brush up the nose to take my attention away from any abdominal discomfort.

"They've put an isolation sign outside the door," Sid says, looking annoyed. "I'm going to the nurses' station to find out what's going on." While he's away, Dr. McCart arrives with two members of her team.

"Hello, Dr. McCart," I say, smiling.

"I'm surprised you recognize me," she laughs, modelling her isolation attire. "Your laparoscopy went well, and we are pleased with what we were able to see. However, a large amount of scar tissue from your first surgery is preventing a good look at your small intestines." She pauses as Sid returns from his mission.

"As I was saying," Dr. McCart continues, "we didn't get a good look at the small intestines, so what I propose is that we go ahead and book you for surgery with the proviso that we start with an examination of the small intestines. If that proves satisfactory, then we would continue with the cytoreductive surgery and HIPEC. How do you feel about that?"

"If you examine the small intestines and don't like what you see, you would just close?"

"Yes."

I make eye contact with Sid, trying to gauge his reaction.

"I've come this far—no turning back now. How long before surgery?" I ask.

"We can book you for September 16."

"That's about six weeks," I mutter.

"It's a Tuesday, but we will admit you on Sunday afternoon and do the pre-surgery prep on Monday."

"Let's do it."

"What I need you to do now is get as strong as you can before you come back to us in September," Dr. McCart instructs. "Will you do that for me?"

"I'll do my best."

"You're going to be with us for a minimum of two weeks after the surgery, then the recovery at home will take a minimum of six months. I know the last few months have weakened you, so you need to regain that strength and more. How are you feeling right now?"

"I feel fine."

"Then I'll have the discharge papers prepared."

Sid puts his arm around me as Dr. McCart leaves. This day hasn't turned out quite like we'd anticipated. Instead of a clear yes or no, we've been handed another maybe. How can I focus on psyching myself up for the super surgery in six weeks when I keep tripping over the maybe?

Our thoughts are interrupted by a nurse entering with discharge instructions and a prescription for pain meds.

Sid moves toward the door. "I'll go to the hotel and get the car while you get dressed."

HESITANT HOPE

"No, don't go. It's such a beautiful day. I'd like to walk. We can take our time and stop at the drugstore on our way."

"Are you sure? It's almost two blocks to the hotel."

"Yes, I'm sure. I can do it."

The sun is deliciously warm on my shoulders as we walk—slowly, carefully.

"What did you find out about my isolation status?"

"I gather they received a complaint."

"Ah yes, the eavesdropping helicopter mom in 1422."

8

SURGERY

You gain strength, courage and confidence by every experience in which you really stop to look fear in the face.

—Eleanor Roosevelt, *You Learn by Living*

The month of August is a gift, an opportunity to savour each day while coaxing my listless body toward renewed vigour. There are no treatments or procedures this month, and I intend to spend as little time as possible thinking about the surgery, at least until September.

Our home away from home at the park has everything I need for comfort. A small space where I feel protected and capable. From the shaded deck, I enjoy bright marigolds Hailey planted in May around the base of a young ash tree. Sandy's canna lilies, in large pots marking the deck corners, display bursts of flaming red. Our picture-perfect view of the lake never grows old.

My goal is to walk my way to fitness on the park trails. At the moment, I can't complete even the smallest circuit, walking but a short distance supported by Sid's steadying arm, then retracing my steps. I have a long way to go, but each day will make a difference. Each day, I'll push a little harder, go a little further. Resistance bands and light weights will help strengthen my upper body.

Our park friends are kind and encouraging, always anxious to hear how I'm doing. When they ask about the upcoming surgery, I try to give them enough information so they'll understand why I believe this treatment is right for me, but I usually realize I've lost them well before my explanation ends. I understand it's complex, and most people are gobsmacked by the invasiveness of the procedure. I'm sure most believe I'm living on borrowed time, reaching for the impossible. I believe, however, that if I can meet the final two criteria and the surgery goes ahead, it will be my salvation.

Gradually, the walks lengthen, and I'm able to increase my pace until a modest cardiac workout is achieved. Heart, lungs, legs and arms—these are the important parts—the parts that will sustain me, pull me back from the brink, get me moving again while my mind is still too foggy from pain meds for my determination to kick in.

Throughout the month, there are many visits from family and friends, all offering their support and best wishes for a good outcome in Toronto. On a particularly beautiful Sunday afternoon, Hailey and Scott arrive with everything needed for a lovely dinner. They busy themselves with the preparation, barbecuing, and cleanup while Grandpa and I relax on the deck. A very special time.

The following weekend finds us in Gatineau helping Samuel celebrate his seventh birthday. Grandchildren are such a treasure. Do I appreciate them more because I'm worried about disappearing from these precious occasions? You bet I do!

In mid-August, Sid subtly explores whether I'm comfortable with him being away for a few hours, then schedules one last shooting range inspection before he must focus on the arrangements for our stay, or more correctly, his stay, in Toronto. The date for the inspection is set, and on Tuesday morning, August 26, I wave goodbye as he drives off. The expression on his face tells me he'd rather not be doing this right now, but we both know I'll be fine—a walk with my book to sit and read, watch the swans, then lunch and an afternoon nap. He'll be back before I know it.

"You'll never guess what I learned today," Sid begins after we're settled on the deck in the late afternoon, each with a tall, cool one.

"Oh?" I can tell this is going to be interesting.

"The range I inspected today is owned by a man named Carman Willows. I happened to mention that his inspection would be my last for this year because I'd be taking you to Toronto in September for a surgery that requires a lengthy convalescence.

"Carman was very interested and wanted to know more about your problem, saying his wife, Emma, had recently been diagnosed with a rare cancer. I gave him the medical term for your illness, and he was flabbergasted, saying that was exactly what Emma had been told.

"Then Carman asked, 'So your wife's going to Toronto for that cowboy surgery?' I didn't know what to say. Cowboy surgery? I told him the surgery you would have is called cytoreductive surgery with HIPEC, and he said, 'That's it—cowboy surgery. It's just plain crazy! Emma doesn't qualify because she's over seventy and her cancer is too advanced.' Our discussion ended when Emma came out of the house carrying a basket of laundry."

"I can't believe it! What incredible odds that you'd happen upon a situation just like mine. How is she doing?"

"She looked good."

We both stare at the lake, lost in thought. The term cowboy surgery threw me, just as it had Sid. Did it make Carman think of bronc-riding at the rodeo—risky, torturous, absurd? Those words certainly described the way I felt in December when it was first offered as a potential option for me. But as horrifying as it seemed, slowly, a metamorphosis began in that dark place of depression and anguish. First as negative curiosity—I don't want to look. Then—do I dare? How could it hurt? I can always turn away. Finally, I'm being drawn like a moth to a flame, to the only thing offering a hand up—a way out of this hell.

Sadness descends as I acknowledge her reality. Mrs. Willows can't experience the incredible life-giving opportunity that is mine—to hold out my hand and accept the hope of a second chance. Up to this point, my attitude toward the upcoming surgery had often been punctuated with fear and reluctance, but suddenly I feel ready to grasp the miracle of modern medicine with both hands.

Once September arrives, Sid begins preparing the RV for an early end to camping season. He also continues to work on a plan for where he'll stay in Toronto while I'm hospitalized. After checking several options in close proximity to the hospital, he discusses his dismay at the cost with our son, Adam, who is an Assistant General Manager for AMICA, a company with upscale retirement residences throughout the province. Adam points out that his company has a complex called the Balmoral Club a few blocks north of Mount Sinai. He's going to contact the manager there to see if something can be arranged. This sounds like it might just be the perfect solution.

With two weeks to go, the surgery is front and centre every waking moment. Even though my commitment is firm, I know the risks, and my mind insists on brooding over worst-case scenarios. My greatest fear is that the exploratory of the small intestines will prove unsatisfactory, and I will wake-up to learn the operation was cancelled. I can't even *image* how I would deal with that.

The possibility, though small, of my demise on the table during the lengthy surgery can't be disregarded, and I'm obsessed with the desire to see my children and grandchildren. With the trip to Toronto for my admission taking place on Sunday, September 14, I arrange a lunchtime get-together for Saturday at The Red George Public House Inc. in Prescott, a convenient midpoint for everyone. Adam, Isabelle, Samuel and William will come from Gatineau, and Hailey will join us from North Gower, near Ottawa. Sandy and Geoff will be enjoying a film festival in Pennsylvania that day, but plan to arrive in Toronto the evening before surgery. I'm so glad Sid won't have to sit through the long stressful day alone.

With only one week to go, the arrangements for Sid's stay at AMICA's Balmoral Club are finalized. He will have a small, one-bedroom suite, and each morning be provided with breakfast and a bag lunch before taking a bus to the hospital. Upon his return in the evening, a meal will be waiting in his refrigerator. A parking space for our car is also included. It's a great package for a reasonable price.

Pauline, a friend who lives in the apartment complex next to ours, is excited to have the pleasure of caring for Max while we're away. It's reassuring to know he'll be visited twice daily, not just for the necessities, but to be brushed and engaged in conversation by a true cat lover. My plants will benefit from her visits as well.

There aren't a lot of things I need to take: house coat and slippers, comfortable neck pillow in the shape of a sleepy white puppy, iPad, hairbrush, toothbrush and paste, moisturizer, clothes for the trip home, and a small glass angel.

My bag is packed.

Saturday is a windy, wet, cold day in Prescott, but the weather cannot dampen my spirits. I'm focused on absorbing every hug, every kiss, every phrase, every peal of laughter as lunch is ordered, served, and savoured.

When the meal is finished, we decide to visit historic Fort Wellington, which is perched on a knoll overlooking the St. Lawrence River at the edge of town. Another precious hour to memorize the love.

On our guided tour, we learn Fort Wellington was a family fort for several years and that the children of the militiamen slept on the floor under their parents' beds.

"No way!" Sam and Will exclaim in disbelief, peering under a bed. Their facial expressions are comical and endearing as they hang on the tour guide's every word.

The tour ends in the arts and craft room where the boys construct militia caps, try on red military tunics, and do the one-eyed squint down the barrel of facsimile rifles.

The time to part has come. Lengthy hugs are shared and many good wishes bestowed.

My only wish is to see them all again.

By Sunday morning, the weather is greatly improved. The drive to Toronto is relaxed and quiet. I'm thankful not to be agonizing over what lies ahead. Perhaps I won't be able to make that claim by tomorrow evening, but at the moment, peace reigns. The first stop of the day will be 155 Balmoral Avenue so Sid can check in, and I can see where he'll be hanging his hat for the next two to three weeks. The staff at the Balmoral Club welcome us warmly, and after telling Sid where to park, show us to his suite. We've no more than made ourselves comfortable after inspecting his new digs, when a staff member carrying an afternoon tea tray taps lightly on the door. I take comfort in knowing he's in a pleasant, friendly place.

Next stop—Mount Sinai Hospital.

HESITANT HOPE

Admissions seem unprepared for my arrival—not the kind of welcome I was expecting. Normally, patients aren't admitted until the morning of surgery, but because I live at a distance, I'd been approved for early admission. All is resolved when an empty bed is found on the orthopaedic floor.

Because medical procedures won't begin until tomorrow, I get permission to leave the hospital for dinner. According to the patient education booklet, this will be my last meal for at least a week.

It means so much to have this couple of hours away from the hospital, a time for the two of us to focus on each other and bask in the love that feeds our courage—perhaps our last opportunity to savour life as we've known it for forty-five good years. In our wildest dreams, we never could have imagined where our forty-sixth year would take us—from planning our next travel destination to discussing preferences for funeral arrangements—from happy family gatherings to choked affairs where artificial smiles are betrayed by a sadness the eyes cannot deny. When dinner ends, we walk slowly, arm in arm, toward the hospital, the setting sun still casting long, chilly shadows in our path.

As expected, my Monday morning breakfast tray contains black coffee and apple juice. Today's pre-surgery routine will involve visits from nurses and doctors, all with questions to ask and examinations to perform. The first visitor is the admissions nurse who collects blood samples, takes swabs, and provides me with two doses of Pico Salax, the first to be taken at 9 a.m., the second at 2 p.m., for the purpose of clearing the digestive tract.

"I want you to drink plenty of clear fluids until midnight," she instructs, "then nothing further." Your surgery is scheduled for 8 a.m., and you need to be ready an hour before."

As one nurse leaves, another enters.

"Mrs. DeVries, I'm here to talk to you about the possibility of an ostomy being part of your surgery tomorrow. I will also be marking your tummy to guide the surgeon as to placement. Do you know what an ostomy is?"

"I know what a colostomy is."

"Good. An ostomy is a surgical procedure to create an opening for waste to be released from the body into a bag. Often, a temporary ostomy is created to allow the bowel to rest and heal without complication, then reversed in three to six months. Sometimes they're permanent. When the procedure is performed on the colon it's called a colostomy, when performed on the small intestines it's called an ileostomy. Not all patients require this procedure, but we need to prepare you in the event it's necessary." She probes and measures until she's satisfied before placing two pea-sized black dots.

"Do you have any questions?"

"If I need to have one I'm sure I'll have questions, but right now I just want to believe it won't be necessary. Will you see me again if the procedure takes place?"

"You can count on it."

The next visit is from Dr. Zeev Friedman who will be my anaesthetist tomorrow. After a brief review of my medical history, he looks down my throat to rule out any problem with the installation of a breathing tube.

"While you're in the ICU, the ventilator will remain in place to allow your body to rest. You'll be given medication so you're able to remain calm while the tube is in place. When you're awake and your breathing is stable, the tube will be removed."

"How long will I be in the ICU?"

"Likely twenty-four to forty-eight hours depending on the extent of your surgery. You'll be under the care of an intensivist, a doctor specializing in intensive care medicine, who is on call around the clock. The nurses in the ICU have special training and take care of only one or two patients, so you'll be monitored closely. Once you're well enough, you'll be moved to the Surgical Step-Down Unit, which is specifically designed for patients still in need of special attention."

I've always been curious about what life is like for doctors and nurses who work in an ICU. Something tells me I'll be in no condition to observe.

"Some bleeding is expected during surgery, but is not normally excessive. I will also be monitoring your heart rate, breathing, and blood pressure, and managing any irregularities."

With all the cutting that's been discussed, I can't imagine not needing a transfusion.

"I'll be placing an epidural catheter in your back first thing in the morning that will provide you with pain control during the operation and for four or five days following. Once you're awake and alert, the nurse will give you a button so you can give yourself pain medication when you need it."

"Can I overdose?"

"No. There's a lock-out period, and if you push your button during a lockout period, no medication will be delivered.

"In addition to the epidural catheter, you'll have several other lines. A cardiac monitor will measure your blood pressure, heart rate, and oxygen. An intravenous line will be inserted in one or both arms to deliver fluids and medication, and an IV will be placed in a large neck vein to help with monitoring while you're in the OR and ICU. A nasogastric tube will be inserted through your nose to your stomach to drain fluid and allow your stomach to rest and recover. Surgical drains will be placed near your incision to help prevent fluid build-up and infection. You'll also have a urinary catheter until you become mobile."

He's so calm, so matter-of-fact. I wish I felt calm.

"Mrs. DeVries? I asked whether you have any questions."

"Sorry. No, your explanations were very clear, and I appreciate knowing what to expect."

"I'll see you first thing in the morning then."

Arriving midmorning, Sid witnesses the beehive of activity and the barrage of information. Between visits by hospital staff, he manages an account of his first overnight at AMICA. I'm amused when he describes how welcoming the other residents—mostly ladies—are to have him join their table at breakfast.

In the late afternoon, Sandy and Geoff breeze in with stories of their weekend away.

"Look at you, sitting there all relaxed and comfortable," Sandy quips. "If it were me, I'd be grabbing my bag and getting out of here."

I smile bashfully at her exaggerated depiction of my courage. Her witticism serves not only to temporarily boost my confidence, but to bring to mind her words from a few days earlier.

"Mom, you know I would do this for you if I could."

Soon, my three musketeers are off to dinner while I continue my clear-liquid diet.

Minutes after Sid returns, Dr. McCart arrives carrying a clipboard.

"You found me!" I exclaim. "I was getting worried."

She smiles as Sid pushes a chair to my bedside, then sits. "I'm glad to see you looking so well. How are you feeling?"

"Good, but anxious."

"That's perfectly understandable. We have a big day ahead of us. I have some papers I need you to sign giving consent."

She explains each section, and I do my best to concentrate, but at this stage I just want to put it all behind me. No more information, no more decisions—let's just do it.

"Do you have any questions for me?" she asks, handing me a pen.

"How many of these surgeries have you done?"

"I checked on that this morning—I must have known you were going to ask. Your surgery will be my ninetieth."

"Do you have any idea how long the surgery will take?"

"It depends on how much disease we find. The maximum length is about twenty hours. If the amount of disease is moderate or minimal, it would of course take less time. Your family can wait in the surgical waiting room on the main floor until it closes at four o'clock, then they can go to the ICU lounge on the eighteenth floor. Your clinical coordinator will provide them with periodic updates."

Turning to Sid, she continues.

"We'll be giving her a lot of fluid during the surgery that will cause swelling in her face and limbs until her body can absorb it, so don't be alarmed when you first see her."

"Thanks for the heads-up."

"Until tomorrow."

When Dr. McCart leaves, Sid takes my hands and looks into my eyes. The mutual fear reflected therein demands a fierce embrace—two drowning souls clinging to the wreckage of kinder days. Whispers of "I love you," slowly calm the tempest.

Sid leaves after reassuring me he'll return early tomorrow.

"I'll see you before you go to the operating room—I promise."

I sit quietly for a few moments. My mind is numb.

A pen clatters to the floor on the other side of the privacy curtain, and a soft voice mutters, "Darn!"

Glad of a diversion, I shuffle around the end of my bed and peer past the curtain where my roommate lies incapacitated, one leg elevated.

"Oh, thank you for coming to my rescue, Dear. My name is Grace. Could you possibly get my pen for me? I should have it on a string."

"Hi, Grace. I'm Helen." I hand Grace her pen.

"Did I hear your doctor correctly? Did she say your surgery could take twenty hours?"

I nod.

"I'm so sorry. What an ordeal you're facing."

"It's all the uncertainty. I hate uncertainty."

"If you don't mind me asking, what are they going to do?"

"That's just it—I don't know. The first hour will be spent determining whether the surgery can be done at all. If they decide to go ahead, every square inch of every organ and every surface in my abdomen will be examined. The organs I can live without will be removed if they show any sign of disease. The organs I can't live without will be cleansed of any visible disease, which may involve removing small segments. Then the entire area will be bathed in heated chemotherapy for ninety minutes. I don't know which organs they'll take or alter. I don't know if I'll need an ostomy. I don't know whether or not all this effort—all this trauma—will result in a cure. And I don't know what my life will be like after recovery—my new normal. It's a nightmare of uncertainty."

"I'm so sorry, Dear."

"I'll be alright Grace. How are you doing?"

"I'm hoping my leg will heal soon so I can go home."

"I hope so too. Sleep well."

Early Tuesday morning, before I have a chance to use the washroom, orderlies are at my door with a gurney.

I slept. Imagine that. I wasn't expecting to.

"Good luck, Dear." Grace calls out, as the nurse helps me onto the gurney.

HESITANT HOPE

Sid, Sandy and Geoff are waiting in the hall and become part of the procession.

When we arrive in the prep area, doctors and nurses swoop in, each with their particular skill set, blending together as paint on a canvas, setting the scene for a potentially life-saving event that wouldn't be possible without them.

While the epidural catheter is being installed, I hear a nurse ask my family to have a seat at the end of the room. I watch until they're seated. The nurse and anesthetist help me lie down, and as the medication begins to flow, I drift into my long, dreamless sleep.

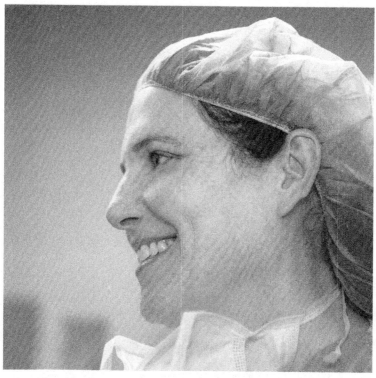

Dr. Andrea McCart in the OR. Photo by Annie Tong, Photographer, Sinai Health System.

9
RECOVERY

Attitude is a little thing that makes a big difference.

—Anonymous

Tuesday, September 16, 2014, approximately 11:30 p.m.:

I'm moving ... wheels wobble, wobble, wobble ...

A young woman dressed in white walks beside me, gripping the rail separating us. She's chewing gum in an open-mouth fashion ... smack, smack, smack ...

Mucous rattles in my windpipe ... I feel like I'm going to choke!

I try to speak, but my throat is blocked.

I struggle and twist ... fighting for my life! My shoulder blades and elbows dig into the hard steel beneath me.

"Stop struggling, Mrs. DeVries. Calm down."

I need to ...

Darkness.

When I flutter toward consciousness again, the hard steel is gone. I feel comfortable and calm. A soft, white mist surrounds me. Two blurry figures are standing by my bed. I think it's Sandy and Geoff. I wonder where Sid is?

A moment later, the ghostly forms turn and move away, joined by a third.

The fog envelops me.

Wednesday, September 17, 2014, midmorning:

The mist has receded. Sid is on my left in silhouette, framed by a wall of windows. The room is awash in natural light. I feel his hand on my shoulder. The steady electronic blip, blip, blip of a monitor echoes my heartbeat.

"There's my strong, brave girl. You came through with flying colours, Sweetheart. You're doing great!"

I manage to focus and meet his happy, relieved gaze. If only I could speak. Why do I still have a tube blocking my throat? Frustration begins to build again. Someone touches my right arm. I turn my head to find Sandy smiling down at me.

"Welcome back."

I blink, wishing I could show her a smile.

From the other side of the bed, a male voice joins the conversation.

"Hello, Mrs. DeVries. I'm Dr. Christian. I'll be taking care of you while you're here in the ICU."

A doctor … this is my chance. I lift my right forearm and pretend to write.

"She wants to say something … I saw a clipboard." Sid moves away for a moment, then hands me a pencil and holds the clipboard in front of me.

HESITANT HOPE

"Get tub out" I scribble in a child-like hand. Will the doctor understand my distress? I must *make* him understand. Drawing a caret after "Get", I scrawl "fucking" above, then drop my hand to the bed. I watch as Sid and the intensivist study my note.

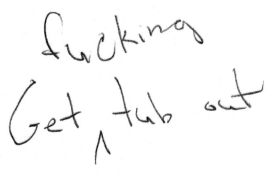

"The tube, she means the tube. Take it out," the doctor instructs.

The nurse moves to the head of my bed, beyond my line of sight, to begin the disconnect process at the source.

"No. Just take it out." he directs. The nurse is at my shoulder reaching for the tube.

It's out! Cough, cough, cough.

"Can you say hello?" the doctor asks.

I form the syllables and expel the air necessary for speech, but my vocal chords won't respond. Going through the motions again, producing a whisper I'm sure only I can hear, seems sufficient to prove my airway is functioning.

I feel such relief. Sleep washes over me again.

Wednesday, September 17, 2014, afternoon:

"How do you feel about sitting up for a few minutes, Mrs. DeVries?" my nurse asks after waking me.

"You want me to get out of bed and sit in a chair?" I ask in disbelief. At this time yesterday, the surgery was still in progress. She can't be serious.

"No, just on the side of the bed. The physiotherapist will be here in a few minutes, and we will both help you."

Minutes later, the process of getting me vertical begins. Some of my lines are attached to a power source at the head of my bed. These are transferred to a portable unit on my IV pole. I have four tubes draining unwanted fluids from my body that must be kept from tangling with each other, as well as the medicinal lines running from the IV pole and the line feeding the epidural catheter. What a daunting task to ensure nothing will be obstructed or disconnected. I can't believe they're going to all this trouble just to move me into a sitting position. Finally, they have everything organized. Bit by bit, the upper portion of the bed is raised. The physiotherapist slides my feet over the edge, then she and the nurse each take a shoulder and ease me into a sitting position. Surprisingly, I feel no stabs of pain—the epidural meds are doing a terrific job.

"You're doing great," the physiotherapist encourages. "How do you feel?"

"Weak."

"That's alright. We won't let go of you."

I know Sid is behind me watching, agonizing, imagining terrible discomfort. I'm glad I can't see the expression on his face.

"How do you feel about standing for a minute. We'll steady you."

They've put so much effort into the preparation, how can I say no? The bed is lowered until my feet touch the floor, then slowly, gently, with a caregiver on each arm, I stand.

"That's it. Now relax for a minute and take a few deep breaths. You're doing great. How does it feel?"

"I'm doing okay," I whisper.

"When you're ready, I'd like you to slide one foot forward."

HESITANT HOPE

I try ... and try ... and try again. My brain is sending the message, but my foot isn't receiving. Why won't it move? My leg is leaden, my muscles unresponsive.

"Try to slide it just a little."

I will it to move, sending the message again and again.

"Take a little break and catch your breath. You're doing great."

This is a taste of what it's like for stroke victims—the struggle to reconnect neural pathways and achieve the movement we take for granted.

With every ounce of strength and determination I can muster, I try once more. This time, my foot moves, sliding forward only an inch or two. It feels so heavy, so awkward.

"Bravo! What an accomplishment! Do you think you can move the other one now?"

It takes only a moment to decide. "No. I'd like to lie down please," I murmur weakly.

"Absolutely. Enough for today."

As they ease me back to bed and reposition my numerous attachments, sleep beckons.

"I'll see you again tomorrow, Mrs. DeVries," the physiotherapist says cheerfully, patting my arm. "You've earned a rest."

Sid kisses my brow as I slip away once more.

Thursday, September 18, 2014:

"Mrs. DeVries, I'm going to sit you up a bit so you can stay awake and talk to us for a few minutes. There are two people here who want to meet you."

"Hello, Mrs. DeVries. I'm Rafael, and this is Olivia. We're from the Surgical Step-Down Unit. Your doctor tells us you're ready to leave Intensive Care and spend a few days with us. Does that sound alright?"

It doesn't seem like I've been here very long. I remember getting the tube out and the visit from the physiotherapist, but …

"How long have I been here?"

"About thirty-six hours."

The ride to the Step-Down Unit is almost as unpleasant as the ride from the OR. I don't remember being too warm while in the ICU, but now I'm sweltering. Is my body still over-heated from the forty-three-degree Celsius chemotherapy? Each time I push the sheet away, the attendant covers me again. At last, in a desperate effort to protect my dignity, he reaches between my legs and pulls the bottom sheet upward to form a tent. Problem solved.

It seems so far. Every doorframe we pass over feels like a speed bump at sixty miles per hour. I'm also blessed to have an orderly-in-training as part of the transfer team who's not yet skilled in navigating corners, and there seem to be so many. By the time we reach our destination, I'm whining like a child.

"Are we there yet? How much further?"

As my stay in the new unit begins, vitals are recorded. The unit is about the size of a ward, but instead of four beds with privacy curtains, there are four small rooms with a monitoring station in the middle.

I'm still much too warm. The vinyl-covered mattress and heavy cotton hospital gown have me damp with perspiration. The level of sedative in my IV is obviously reduced, making me more alert and aware of discomfort. The patient-controlled analgesia pump that allows me to give myself pain medication at the push of a button is now at my fingertips. My resistance to using it will no doubt be overcome quickly when I become too uncomfortable.

To check on the effectiveness of the nerve block still being delivered by the epidural catheter, the nurse touches me with an ice cube at several points on my chest and abdomen. The only areas that register the sensation of cold are near my shoulders and at my groin. My blood pressure, which was monitored minute to minute by the arterial line, is now being recorded by an arm cuff that inflates every half hour. Sid was baffled by erratic readings displayed on the electronic panel over my bed during the thirty-six hours in the ICU. Hopefully, it will stabilize soon—the cuff delivers quite a pinch when inflated.

My nurse for the evening shift is a handsome male of Latin American origin.

"Would you like a sponge bath this evening, Mrs. DeVries?"

This young man could be my son, my grandson even. I look at him without speaking.

"It might help you sleep," he offers encouragingly.

A sponge bath *would* feel wonderful. Can I set timidity aside? Female nurses have always bathed male patients. He is a nurse after all.

"Yes, it would help me sleep."

He moves about my small space closing curtains, both to the nurses' station and to the world at large. After assembling a large metal basin, soap and a stack of washcloths and towels, we're ready to begin. Will I be sorry I agreed to this?

Towels are placed discreetly over my chest and pelvic area as my gown is gently removed. He bathes one arm, then dips a fresh washcloth before moving to the other. When my arms are finished, he hands a warm, moist cloth to me and asks me to do my face and neck while he washes my mid-section, never once returning a soiled cloth to the basin. Before beginning my lower extremities, he hands me another cloth to use on my chest, adding that he can assist if I have difficulty. This is the part I was worried about, so now I can relax. A fresh gown is slipped over my arms and the protective towels removed. His attention then turns to my back and changing the bottom sheet. These steps are accomplished with the help of a towel rolled from the side to form a cylinder. This is placed behind me, after I've been turned on my side with the help of a second nurse, and holds me in place until one side is bathed. Then, with a gentle push from the other side, I'm effortlessly flipped via the soft fulcrum under my spine. The clean bottom sheet gradually replaces the soiled one as I'm turned. Technique is everything.

The positive effects of the sponge bath are more psychological than physical. I'm soon wishing I could be free of the vinyl beneath me and the coverings above—hot and clammy again. I poke the button on the PCA hoping an extra shot of pain meds will allow me to sleep.

Sometime during the night, I awake in agony.

"My hands hurt," I moan to the doctor on my right. Several figures in white smocks are gathered around my bed. My nurse enters with a hypo, the contents of which he injects into my left arm, causing me to slide into a pain-free slumber while the professionals do their work.

Friday, September 19, 2014:

"Breathe deeply, Mrs. DeVries. We need you to breathe deeply." Morning sunlight floods my room. I'm sitting upright.

"I *am* breathing. This is how I normally breathe. I'm not a deep breather."

"You need to breathe deeply. You don't have enough oxygen in your blood, and we don't want to put you back on oxygen."

Of all the lines attached to me in the ICU, I didn't notice the oxygen—I'm sure there were many things I didn't notice. The tube in my throat garnered most of my attention.

I can't see a monitor, but I've obviously being ratted out by some electronic gizmo.

How long has it been, early childhood I suspect, since I've been comfortable not knowing what time it is? For the past two days, I've been content simply identifying day and night. I know it's daytime if Sid is sitting by my bed and I see light at the window. If I'm alone, and light shines only from the nurses' station, it's nighttime. Daylight has broken—he's on his way. I'll ask him to bring my watch tomorrow.

"How was your night?" Sid asks, still recovering from his sprint from the subway station.

"I guess I had a breathing problem at some point. They raised the head of my bed and kept ordering me to breathe deeply. Very annoying."

Dr. McCart is on rounds, followed by several colleagues.

"Good morning, Mrs. DeVries. How are you doing?"

"I'm not sure. I don't think I'm a very good patient."

Dr. McCart turns toward the nurses' station and inquires loudly, "Who told Mrs. DeVries she isn't a very good patient?"

"I made quite a fuss during the night. I don't know what was wrong."

"It's called hypoxemia, an abnormally low level of oxygen in the blood, and it's not uncommon after a major surgery like you've had. We're getting it under control with your help. How are you doing otherwise?"

"My mouth is dry, and my throat hurts every time I swallow."

"There are swabs that will help with the dryness, and we'll check to see if the NG tube can come out. The physiotherapist will see you again today—we need to get you walking."

"How did the surgery go?"

"As you know, our plan was to begin with a thorough examination of the small intestines. We found a considerable amount of disease at the terminal ileum close to the large bowel, however, we felt that everything we saw was completely resectable while still leaving you with a significant amount of small bowel, so we decided to go ahead with the operation."

"That would have been when the surgical coordinator called me with an update," Sid interjects.

"We removed the omentum first, then moved to your pelvis where the majority of your disease was. We knew the right ovary and the uterus were involved, but on closer inspection determined there was disease on the bladder and the wall of the right lower quadrant. The ovary and the uterus were removed first, then we stripped the bladder peritoneum as well as both the right and left lower quadrant peritoneums."

"I must have lost a lot of blood."

"Only about five hundred millilitres—not enough to require a transfusion. The use of cautery helps reduce the amount of bleeding.

"The work on the small bowel involved removing approximately two feet, plus a small portion of the colon. The lesser omentum was also removed, and when we moved the liver we found soft disease on the diaphragm wall, so the right diaphragm peritoneum was stripped."

"There was no disease on my liver?"

"No, and your spleen and stomach were also clear. We took a good look at everything again, then prepared you for the chemotherapy."

"What does that involve?"

"Two tubes are placed, one on each side of your chest, for the inflow, and a catheter is placed in the pelvis for the outflow. The abdomen is closed with sutures, and the tube sites packed with Vaseline gauze. The chemotherapy, Mitomycin-C, is circulated by pumps through a heater to keep the temperature at forty-three degrees Celsius before entering your body. As the heated wash circulates for ninety minutes, we massage your abdomen to ensure no area is untouched by the chemotherapy. After ninety minutes, the abdomen is rinsed thoroughly and reopened so we can remove the tubes and reconnect the small intestine to the colon."

"Why did you leave that until after the HIPEC wash?"

"To ensure that the margins of both organs were fully exposed to the chemotherapy."

"Now you're ready for the final closing?"

"Yes, and after we close, there are still drains to be installed. It was about 11:30 p.m. when we sent you to the ICU.

While Dr. McCart and I were talking, my nurse repositioned the NG collection pouch so the drainage from my stomach would stop. Within minutes of Dr. McCart's departure, I'm vomiting. Obviously, the nasogastric tube is still necessary. Perhaps I can swallow less often—good luck with that.

My nurse for the day is a well-seasoned matron who provides a thorough bathing.

"Would it be possible to have my hair washed?"

"I'll check for you," she replies, leaving the room. In a moment, she returns. "We have to wait until the central line is removed from your neck. Maybe by then you'll be able to use the shower." The sponge bath is refreshing, but having my hair shampooed would be the icing on the cake.

Soon.

The preparation required of the physiotherapist to get me moving is still intricate. In an e-mail Sid sent after surgery, he described me and my network of tubes as looking like the space shuttle on launch day. The space shuttle analogy still applies. I manage five or six short steps from my bed to the door of my room.

Saturday, September 20, 2014:

I had a dream last night. A sparkling glass bowl filled with mouth-watering fruit—scarlet strawberries, indigo blueberries, shimmering blackberries, misty-green grapes, and fuzzy peaches—was floating above the foot of my bed. My body has complained in many ways during the past week, but hunger is not a sensation I've noticed. It would seem, however, that my subconscious has noted the deprivation. Fresh fruit atop my morning cereal—that's how I like to start my day.

Soon.

Two lovely surprises serve to reconnect me with the world beyond Mount Sinai. First, a beautiful floral arrangement is delivered from Sid's colleagues at the Chief Firearms Office, then a visit from Mike and Carol Quilty, friends from Sid's years with the O.P.P.

Special units like the ICU and Surgical Step-Down are protective bubbles where patients in critical condition receive the best care available. While there, your world is small and you're aware of little. What you *are* aware of leads you to believe you're the centre of this universe. But no, people from *out there* have sent me flowers, people from *out there* have come to visit. I have survived!

The world beyond this hospital is calling me back, demanding I resolve to return as a full partner.

Soon.

My half-hour with the physiotherapist gets me to the door of my room, then part way through the nurses' station attempting a breakaway to the hall. Not quite—perhaps tomorrow. Each day, little improvements—baby steps. When the nurse does her regular check with the ice cube, the area of non-response is quite small. The epidural nerve block will soon be nonexistent.

Two things are not improving. With each swallow, the NG tube continues to irritate an already bruised throat. My complaints are met with, "If we take it out too soon, we'll only have to put it back." My discomfort with the blood pressure cuff is worsening. The nurse tries it on my leg, but that is even more painful. These issues are minor compared to the overall picture, but distressing nonetheless.

Sunday, September 21, 2014:

The physiotherapist is back—this lady has the patience of Job. Before our session ends, I manage a few steps into the hallway before returning to my bed exhausted, but proud of my accomplishment. Getting into the hallway reinforces my sense of returning to the real world—other patients, visitors, nurses, and doctors going about their duties, duties that have nothing to do with me. This is my fourth day in the Step-Down Unit.

Monday, September 22, 2014:

Today is Sid's birthday. I have no card or gift for him. That's a first, and it makes me sad.

The medical team arrives early to assess my progress, and after reviewing my chart and asking a few questions decides I'm ready for discharge to the floor.

"While you're under general nursing care, your pain will be managed with analgesia given by mouth, so we'll be removing the epidural catheter this morning. We'll also remove the central line from your neck and the blood pressure cuff."

Yeah! Three less appendages, no more ice-cube checks, and I can finally wash my hair.

One thing I won't be free of is the twice-daily injection of Heparin, a drug designed to assist in the prevention of blood clots after surgery. I dread seeing the nurse approach with that nasty, stinging-bee of a shot. One more good-for-you experience one wishes wasn't necessary.

The new room is a semi-private with my bed being the one closest to the door and the bathroom. My roommate, who I would guess is about ten years my junior, appears to be well into her recovery. She's wearing an IV nutrition pouch on a shoulder strap, however, which indicates solid food is not yet tolerated.

One week post-surgery and I'm finally on my own—no more minute-to-minute monitoring. A call button is how I'll get assistance, but with Sid close by during the day, I should only need to summon the nurse when pain meds are required. The physiotherapist won't be seeing me again, and I've been instructed to walk the halls as much as possible. In the evening, my niece Debbie and nephew Mike surprise me with a visit and flowers.

HESITANT HOPE

Tuesday, September 23, 2014:

One more hanger-on bites the dust. The Foley catheter is removed, giving me another option for exercise—trips to the bathroom. I can finally have a shower. Thankfully, the shower room is large, with a chair, hand rails, and adjustable-height shower heads. I hope I get through this before exhaustion strikes. There are still two drain lines attached to my belly and the nasogastric tube coming from my nose. This is complicated. Maybe I should have asked Sid to come in with me—an extra pair of hands would help. Don't panic. Just take your time. This is what you've been waiting for, so don't spoil it. I'm very tired by the time I finish, but it feels wonderful to have clean hair at last.

Geoff is in Toronto on his days off this week. He sits with me for a couple of hours in the afternoon, giving Sid a much-needed break. He reads to me from Margaret Laurence's *The Stone Angel*, which I brought from home but find I'm too uncomfortable to read. Geoff's expressive voice makes the text riveting, and I'm enjoying the story very much. I'll be sorry when he goes home. He'll visit his sister tonight, then return tomorrow to chat and read again.

My roommate is fully dressed.

"I'm breaking out for the afternoon," she chirps, passing my bed on her way out the door.

That's perfectly fine with me—if only her doctor would give her a full discharge, I'd be happy. My problem with being too warm isn't going away. I'm becoming more uncomfortable as each hour passes. There is air conditioning, but my roommate has covered the vents, which are on her side of the room, with enough towels to completely block the flow of cool air. Sid talks to one of the staff, and shortly thereafter a maintenance worker arrives to check the thermostat. To his surprise, he finds it set at over eighty degrees Fahrenheit. He lowers the setting to a more reasonable seventy-four, and in a few hours the room is comfortable again.

When the nurse checks the collection container in the bathroom at the end of the day, she seems concerned about the minimal urine output. She rushes from my room and returns minutes later with a portable ultrasound machine. My bladder experienced significant trauma during surgery because tumour tissue needed to be removed from the surface. All seems to be well, however, as doctors are not summoned.

Wednesday, September 24, 2014:

What a comfortable sleep I had last night. Unfortunately, my comfort is short-lived.

"Who got to you?"

I'm hearing one side of a telephone conversation through the privacy curtain.

As the day passes, the temperature again builds to a suffocating level. There will be little sleep tonight. She must have an accomplice who reset the thermostat while I was out of the room for a walk. Who is this frozen witch, and what are her connections?

When her husband arrives, she isn't long asking, "Did you find the gift I left for you yesterday?"

"No."

"I left it under the covers on your side of the bed."

She's been having frequent visits from a nurse whose concerns seem different from the regular nursing staff. While my nurse injects me with my Heparin shot around 8 p.m., her nurse is instructing the husband to "take this a half to one hour before, if you need to." My nurse pulls the curtain aside just enough for a peek, then laughs, "It doesn't look like it'll be necessary."

Never would I have imagined that being witness to a sex therapy session in the next bed would be part of my recovery.

I've been asking for pain relief on a regular basis, but I'm having trouble distinguishing pain related to surgery from pain caused by intestinal gas which the meds won't help. Then there's the discomfort resulting from the excessive heat, and the frustration from being made party to my neighbour's private life. I know I'm not ready to go home, but right now I'm wishing I were anywhere but here. I try sitting in a chair, adjusting my hospital gown to cover as little as modesty will allow. I'm tired and need to sleep, but my bed is hot and my pillow is hot.

The room lights are off, but a fluorescent invasion streams through the open door. As I sit staring at the floor, it begins to undulate like waves at the beach. I watch for a moment, amused, then avert my eyes, thinking they'll clear, but instead, a polar bear is staring at me from my bed. While I gawk at him in disbelief, his leathery black nose becomes an open space. Dropping my gaze back to the floor, it now seems a breeze is lifting it, like a patio rug on a windy day.

"This is definitely not a good thing, Helen—best back off on the pain meds," I mutter.

The last few minutes have taken a disturbing toll. I'm feeling alone and vulnerable as I stumble back to bed, tears rolling down my cheeks. I must sleep now so this night will pass and Sid will be here taking care of me again. The temperature of my bed and pillow are more comfortable, and I fall into a fitful sleep that seems but a continuation of the circumstances that forced me from the chair. In my nightmare, I'm outside, snow blowing around me. I'm hugging my hospital gown to my body. It's so cold. There's a door, but if I move the bear will see me.

"What are you doing, Mrs. DeVries?" my nurse asks.

Where did she come from? I've been jerked from my private hell to find I'm sitting on the side of my bed tugging on my gown.

"What are you trying to do?"

I can't tell her about the bear—she'll think I'm crazy.

"I need to go to the bathroom."

"Do you need my help?"

"No, I think I can manage."

Thursday, September 25, 2014:

What a relief to find Sid sitting at my bedside when I open my eyes. "I'm so glad you're here," I whisper when he hugs me.

"Did you have a good night?"

"Give me a couple minutes to freshen up, then we'll take a walk—it's cooler in the hall."

After unloading my pathetic tale while pushing my IV pole up and down the corridor several times, I'm settling back to bed when a lady dressed in a business suit greets us. She explains that it's her role to help patients with any problems they might be experiencing.

"How is everything going with you, Mrs. DeVries?"

Sid stands and motions her into the hallway so I won't have to explain within earshot of my roommate.

"I've filled her in. We'll wait and see what she can do," he says when he returns.

In less than an hour, a nurse enters. "You want to move to a different room?"

"Yes, I would like to move to a cooler room."

"I think we've found a place that will work for you. Jill likes it cooler as well."

The move takes only minutes, and I'm very, very grateful for the change.

Jill is a sweet, young lady about twenty years of age. Intestinal problems have plagued her since childhood, and she received treatment at Sick Kids until she was eighteen. Her mother stays with her day and night, and a brief, private conversation with her made us aware that Jill's future is bleak. The window sills in the large corner room are loaded with floral tributes. The temperature is perfect—I am so comfortable here.

Friday, September 26, 2014:

When the doctor visits this morning, I'm over the moon to hear the NG tube and the remaining IV lines will be removed today, and I can begin a liquid diet. I have come a long way. A lovely bouquet arrives from Betty Ann, giving my over-the-bed table a cheerful splash.

Saturday, September 27, 2014:

The return of mealtime adds new structure to my day. Coffee, tea, milk, juice, porridge, broth, jello, and puddings are welcome choices on my tray. An afternoon visit from Mary Ann and Glenn is an enjoyable interlude. During the evening, many relatives and friends gather to spend time with Jill. Could it be a birthday celebration? After everyone leaves, she has a painful night.

Sunday, September 28, 2014:

Adam and family arrive from Gatineau, Quebec, and I'm so happy to see them. After hugs and kisses, little four-year-old William has a question for Grandma.

"Grandma, is this where you live now?"

The question is asked in a sweet, gentle manner that causes my heart to burst with love, but at the same time, I feel a stab of regret that my darling little grandson is concerned about how his relationship with Grandma might be changing.

"Grandma is here to get better, William. Then I'm going home."

We spend time walking and talking together, visiting the gift shop on the ground floor. The visitors' lounge across the hall from my room helps keep the boys entertained. They stay for the afternoon, then begin the long drive home, which will take about five hours.

Small sips of liquid are going down well. I can't get excited about the coffee though— it's the same colour as the liquid the nasogastric tube was draining from my stomach.

Monday, September 29, 2014:

Early rounds by the gastrointestinal team start my day with a blast. After the usual, "How are you feeling?" the next question is, "Would you like to go home today?"

"Yes, I would like that very much!"

"Then we'll have your drains and staples removed, and the pharmacist will be in to see you with pain meds and instructions on managing any pain you may still have."

Having the staples removed isn't of concern because I'd had a painless experience in November after the first surgery. But the drains? That has me worried—I don't know what to expect.

As soon as they leave, I'm on the phone to Sid giving him the good news.

"They're discharging me today!"

"You're kidding! Wow, I never expected that. I'll have to get signed out here and bring the car. How long do you think it'll be before you're ready?"

"Two hours should do it."

"I'll be there as soon as I can."

Removing the staples takes about half an hour. I try to count them when the nurse is finished, but find it too tedious, stopping at seventy, a little over half. The drains are ripped out, each with a rapid, forceful pull that leaves me gasping.

The pharmacist delivers a supply of oxycodone, sternly advising me to switch to Tylenol as soon as possible.

While waiting for Sid, I peek around Jill's curtain hoping to wish her well before I leave. The sweet child is sleeping, and I don't have the heart to wake her.

When Sid arrives, he gathers my things and we make our way to the nurses' station to checkout, thanking everyone for their excellent care. Jill's mother is there, so we are able to offer her our best wishes.

Again, I feel very fortunate.

10
REFLECTING ON A NEW BEGINNING

"Hope" is the thing with feathers—
That perches in the soul—
And sings the tune without the words—
And never stops—at all—

—Emily Dickinson

The battle plan laid before me in December 2013 didn't exist a decade ago. Yet here I am, the fortunate and thankful beneficiary of another amazing advance in cancer treatment. The timing couldn't have been better. After ten long months of rigorous compliance, I'm going home to heal.

Returning home has always been a sweet experience for me, an opportunity to see with fresh eyes my ever-evolving Eden. Several years ago, on a night flight home from a European holiday, I remember designing a photo gallery for a room-size hallway in our home that deserved a fresh focus. After a three-month winter getaway in the south, I was eager to reorganize every cupboard and closet. How crazy is that? This time, my goal is to heal. This return is like no other—I've crossed the Jordan. I want to welcome each day, each week, each month, and the potential they offer.

"What was the day of the operation like for you?" I ask Sid as we near our destination.

"I was fairly calm for the first couple of hours," he began.

"I'm sure having Sandy and Geoff with you helped."

"It did. A call came from the surgical coordinator at about 11 a.m. to say the exploratory was finished, and they were proceeding with the cytoreductive procedure. It was a huge relief to know they were going ahead, but now it hit home just how long this day was going to be."

"I remember Dr. McCart brushing off my concerns about the length of the surgery by saying, 'Don't worry, you'll be sleeping the entire time,'" I chuckle.

"I left the hospital with Sandy and Geoff around noon to get some lunch, and then we spent some time at their hotel. I knew the hospital could reach me on my cell, but by mid-afternoon I became anxious and insisted we return to the hospital. I needed to be close to you. There was a pub off the main lobby—we had a drink before heading back.

"As the afternoon wore on, I became more restless and began to pace. I couldn't stop thinking about what they were doing—the lengthy incision, lifting everything out, examining inch by inch, cutting, cutting, cutting. The longer I waited, the more I worried that something had gone wrong—that the next call would bring bad news.

"By 5 p.m., I was frantic.

"Finally, the phone rang. The surgery was complete, and the HIPEC treatment was about to begin. It was just after 7 p.m. when I looked at my watch."

"Which meant you still had another three or four hours to go."

"We moved to the ICU waiting room where Dr. McCart said she'd meet with us. It was close to midnight when she came to tell us you were on your way. She was pleased with the outcome and confident that all the visible tumour tissue had been removed.

Fortunately, the burden of disease was less than expected making the time in the OR a modest fourteen hours. She warned us you might not be conscious when we saw you, and that you'd be very swollen due to the amount of fluids given. She also cautioned us regarding the number of lines and tubes attached to you.

"After the ICU staff had you settled, we were able to see you for a few minutes, and yes, you were very swollen—Sandy said she wouldn't have recognized you had she not been given a heads-up. Then, reluctantly, but also with great relief, we left to find some dinner."

"I vaguely remember misty figures moving around my bed in the ICU."

It is, indeed, wonderful to be home. The apprehension I felt on the day we departed—wondering what my return was going to look like—is no longer relevant. Max is glad to see me and wastes no time joining me on the bed, settling beside me with his chin on my chest to keep watch. Sid is unpacking my travel bag and hands me *The Stone Angel*. The pleasant memory of Geoff's voice and an absorbing tale are all that remain—recall of the plot is nowhere to be found.

Sandy and Adam have each arranged a week off to help with my care, but because we'd anticipated a three week stay in hospital rather than the surprising two, our scheduling is askew by one week. Betty Ann is happy to fill in until Adam arrives and sets to work preparing meals of soft, lightly-seasoned food we think I'll be able to digest easily. My instructions are to eat whatever I want, but in small quantities.

It's not going well. It's only my second day home, and everything I put in my mouth seems to go straight through in a matter of minutes. We try making my diet bland, even resorting to mostly fluids. We eliminate juices due to the sugar content and read labels to avoid sugar and sugar substitutes, all of which act as softeners. I try commercial meal-in-a-bottle drinks. The BRAT diet is also given a spin because foods such as bananas, rice, applesauce, and toast have a binding affect. Nothing seems to make a difference. Thanksgiving is just around the corner, and Adam is planning a special dinner to celebrate the successful completion of my treatment. Alas, my time is divided between the bathroom and bedroom on Thanksgiving Day. I'm not able to join in the feasting, but everyone gathers around in the bedroom before parting, which tempers my disappointment somewhat. Is this how it's going to be? Is this my new normal? Give it time—it's only been four weeks.

At a visit with Dr. Robinson on October 16, one month post-surgery to review my digestive problems, the bottom line seems to be that my symptoms are not surprising considering the removal of a portion of the small intestine plus the added irritation of the heated chemotherapy. She suggests that ceasing the oxycodone meds could also be a factor. As a matter of caution, I'm asked to provide samples for testing to rule out C. difficile.

I'm scheduled to return to Toronto for my post-surgery checkup on Friday, October 24. To say I'm worried is an understatement. How can I possibly make this trip when I can't get through one hour without a bathroom? My best bet is to fast on the 24th, and I will also try to familiarize myself with every rest stop along the highway.

As is often the case, my worries loom larger than life itself. We make the trip without incident. Dr. McCart is pleased to see the incision is healing well and that I'm experiencing no abdominal pain or distension. We discuss foods I should avoid to help get the persistent diarrhea under control, in particular, raw fruits and vegetables. So much for my fruit-bowl dream. Imodium is prescribed to provide additional assurance when I need to travel. A baseline CT scan will be ordered, and I'm to return in two months.

My progress is slow and my accomplishments small. Since September 16, I've been sleeping only on my back. Every few days, I try rolling to one side or the other, but the discomfort is always unbearable, and I quickly relent. Perhaps next time. One small triumph occurs when I stop in my tracks at the sight of a stooped old woman shuffling past mirrored closet doors in our apartment. I'm obviously favouring my incision, and even in bed I sleep with two or more pillows under my head and shoulders. It's time to straighten my spine and stand tall again.

In mid-November, two months post-surgery, I decide to return to Tai Chi class at the Seniors' Centre, as I feel the slow, gentle movements of the set will help rebuild strength and balance. I find it necessary to sit occasionally, but the fact that I'm able to participate is colossal. Attending class also gets me driving again, only a few blocks, but it feels good to regain some independence. It's been a year since I last sat behind the wheel.

Independence. Nations covet it and fight wars to defend it. Youth clamour tirelessly for it. At the opposite end of the lifecycle, senescent men and women often experience anxiety and depression as their lives slide unapologetically into physical and mental decline. Experiencing long-term illness is yet another way to lose autonomy. As much as I needed and appreciated the excellent care Sid provided over the past year, I am slowly regaining my strength, and with it, the desire to do things for myself. If I say, "I think I'll make a cup of tea," he seems to hear "I think I'd like a cup of tea," and springs into action. I need to resume at least partial control of my life—feel competent again. Sid, however, is content in the caregiver role and fails to understand my frustration. I'm sure some would consider this an ideal circumstance. For me, it's a struggle. I wonder if his compulsion to meet my every need stems from his feeling of powerlessness at not being able to solve the bigger problem?

On December 7, my sixty-fifth birthday, Sid and I are among forty other couples celebrating at a Christmas dinner party in our apartment building. The surprise gift of a lovely bouquet and a spirited rendition of "Happy Birthday" make the evening particularly memorable. This is the first time since the operation that I've attempted to eat a complete meal at one sitting, ignoring the doctor's advice about small quantities. My stomach is not happy. Thankfully, I'm able to return to our apartment without interrupting Sid's evening, where I walk the floor until the discomfort passes. Not only is my system not ready to digest salad, but adding dessert immediately after the main course was definitely poor judgment. When we gather at Sandy's for our family Christmas, I'm a little wiser.

Once Christmas celebrations are over, my thoughts target the next step in my follow-up. My first post-op CT scan, which will be used as a baseline for comparison of future scans, is set for January 6, 2015. Until now, I've been calm and relaxed, understanding that the purpose of this scan is not diagnostic. An unwelcome guest, however, slips in through the back door—anxiety. In spite of a good understanding of where I am at slightly over three-months post-surgery with healing still underway, my mind insists on wandering shadowy paths of morbid imaginings. Logic will take a back seat until I receive assurances from Dr. McCart at my clinic appointment on January 16.

As common sense would dictate, the recent scan shows nothing surprising. I'm able to report a small improvement in the functioning of my digestive tract and a gradual increase in my strength and stamina since my last visit.

HESITANT HOPE

The anxiety related to uncertainties that came with the territory when I decided to pursue cytoreductive surgery with HIPEC were numerous and nerve-wracking. Would I be successful in meeting the qualifying criteria? Would I make a complete recovery, or would I need to adapt to a new normal? Would my disease return in a short period of time, would I be cured, or would the end result be somewhere in between? Through it all, I've held fast to the belief that only one thing could be worse than all the uncertainty—certain death.

I must admit, however, that even though I'm in awe of the miracle of modern medicine that repaired my broken body and restored my hope of a future, there are moments every now and again when I wonder whether the decision to accept treatment was the right one, considering some of life's dilemmas that spur bouts of melancholy. I realize that those who've been spared the bitter wine of depression may scoff at such a notion, but an old adage describes it well: *To those who know, no explanation is necessary, to those who don't know, no explanation is sufficient.*

As my energy slowly returns, I look for ways to make small contributions to the household routine. I've always enjoyed laundry day and feel ready to help by stripping the bed. Clean, crisp linens are one of life's little pleasures. While shaking the pillow from its case on Sid's side, tears of love and thankfulness begin falling for the man who lays his tired head here night after night—a man who gives so much and asks so little. As I lift a fitted corner from the mattress, I sense longing and restraint entwined. How can I tell him I'm afraid?

Only one scar can be seen, but frequently I wake suddenly, my heart pounding, my mind reeling with fearful thoughts and images of infiltration, violation. Yes, I agreed to the surgical procedure, but the invasiveness of it now haunts me. During the period leading up to surgery, I was blessed with a concentrated focus that saw only a positive outcome and cloaked the frightening realities.

I'm seeing flashes of my draped, defenseless body; a gaping, empty abdomen; a raw, bloody cavity stripped of peritoneal lining; resection of intestines; severing of omentum; peeling of bladder peritoneum; the extrication of a spent uterus and ovary—necessitating repairs to a vaginal canal now devoid of connecting tissue.

Now that my appointment in Toronto is behind us, Sid prepares for cataract surgery. Once his recovery is complete, we are both looking forward to five weeks in the south for a much-needed break from all things medical. I'm glad I've been driving again, as now Sid needs to be chauffeured periodically, and I am more than happy to oblige.

While south, we meet dear friends from home who are travelling with their RV. Our relationship with Fred and Mary spans many years. Sid and Fred were childhood pals, and each stood as best man for the other when Cupid called. They've been particularly supportive over the past year because Mary's been dealing with metastatic breast cancer and understands my dilemma in a way only another cancer patient can. She's managing well with continued treatment, but knows she will succumb. Cancer has spread to her bones.

I spend as much time as possible at the beach, watching and listening to the ocean—so good for the soul. Sometimes the rhythm of the surf lulls me into a peaceful place where cares are not allowed. On other occasions, the same waves inspire one to explore the meaning of life with its many twists and turns. I often find myself contemplating a question asked by a member of my writers' group.

"How has this experience changed you?"

HESITANT HOPE

The question seems to haunt me, no doubt because I'm having trouble discovering the truth. Yet not to be a different person after such a traumatic few months seems unlikely.

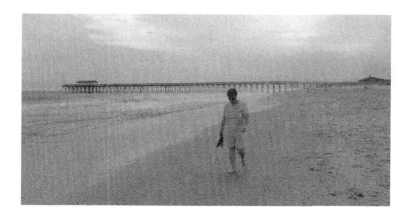

Not long after my crushing diagnosis, but before hope appeared on the horizon, I was walking in the downtown area where I saw a homeless man sitting on the sidewalk. I remember being surprised that I didn't feel the need to turn my head away or give him a wide berth. Have I developed a stronger bond with all mankind? Have I stopped being fearful of those who are different? I've also noticed I'm not as concerned about dust on the furniture, or toys on the floor when my grandsons visit. Is it possible I've become kinder with myself? It will be interesting to see if these changes remain or gradually fade with my scar.

The beach is also a great place to walk, particularly at low tide when there's a wide band of firm, damp sand to the water's edge. When we arrived in Myrtle Beach, I found the flight of stairs to our second-floor suite challenging, but by the time we pack for home, I do them easily. It feels great to be getting stronger and more energetic.

One of the difficulties I'm just beginning to experience, however, is a feeling of loneliness, or perhaps abandonment is a better word. I know it makes me sound like a spoiled child, but believe me, it's real. From the moment testing begins, through diagnosis, chemotherapy, surgeries, and initial recovery, the attention from doctors, nurses, family, and friends is constant and abundant. Once the crisis has passed, the need for medical care is greatly reduced, and family and friends have reasonably returned to a lower alert level. This is all very sensible and natural, but it means managing the continuing struggles of recovery without the attention and encouragement I've become addicted to. It really is the perfect time to reconstruct my life—the life I thought was over.

Before my illness, I dabbled in creative writing and photography. As my recovery progresses, I feel inspired to write about my unusual medical journey—to share the patient's perspective. I've noticed many people shy away from conversation with the critically ill, not knowing what to say or fearing they'll say something inappropriate. I'm hoping the people who read my story will understand that I am still the same person I was, albeit with a new, unpalatable circumstance.

As for photography, I have little desire to spend much time behind the lens. My objective is to be fully present in every situation rather than checking shutter speed and aperture setting or changing lenses.

When we return home from Myrtle Beach in early April, the next scan is only a week away. Try as I might to remain calm, anxiety builds. I tell myself worrying is a waste of time and will make no difference in the results, but I worry anyway. We try to keep busy, but I know I'm not myself—impatient, irritable, not sleeping well. I know how happy and relieved I'll be if the results are good, but what if …? No, no, no … don't go there. I'll daydream about our Alaskan cruise in July.

This follow-up appointment is with Dr. Biagi in Kingston on April 14, 2015, and he's obviously pleased to see me looking well. He is not pleased, however, to learn I'm still experiencing neuropathy in my hands and feet and expresses regret that this is the case. Then he advises that no worrisome changes were seen in the latest scan. I'm overjoyed!

"This is a good result, but we need to wait for a few more scans before we celebrate," he cautions.

But we *do* celebrate on April 20, our forty-seventh wedding anniversary. I may still have a long way to go, but I've come so far.

The following week, an invitation arrives from Fred and Mary asking us to join them at the Royal Coachmen in Napanee for a celebration of their forty-fifth wedding anniversary. Family and friends gather on May 30, to share memories and a delicious meal. Mary has lost a lot of weight over the last couple of months, and her voice is weak and raspy as she speaks to her loved ones. How much longer?

Within two weeks, Mary is admitted to hospital and passes away on June 24, 2015. This is the third friend to be taken by cancer in the past year.

But life goes on.

Open suitcases wait expectantly on the bedroom floor while we debate how best to outfit ourselves for every type of weather without taking our entire closet. Cruise brochures for Alaska tempt travelers to "see one of nature's last frontiers," and we look forward to reveling in the majesty of glaciers, mountains, rivers, and forests after our flights on July 15, first to Vancouver, then to Anchorage. There is nothing like the awesome handiwork of Mother Nature to put things in perspective—to make one feel small and insignificant yet ever so privileged to be a part of it all. Like the fireweed that bathes Alaska in vibrant red from June through September, we are a vital and beautiful part of the summer landscape, but as winter approaches, colours fade and growth gives way to decay, laying the groundwork for new life when the spring sun again warms the Arctic tundra.

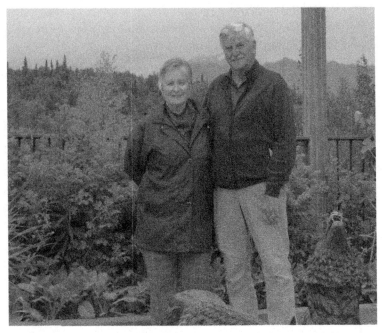

When we disembark in Ketchikan, Sid and I board a bus that takes us to Totem Bight State Historical Park. This is an important stop for me because I've be in awe of totem poles since childhood. One's imagination runs free in the quest to reclaim stories of past lives as told through the symbolic carving on each pole. I wish I could stay longer, but a chilling rain and a bus schedule are making demands.

Our tour of choice in Juneau is the DIPAC Macaulay Salmon Hatchery where millions of fingerlings are released each spring.

HESITANT HOPE

The survivors will return as adults, fighting their way up the manmade fish ladder into the hatchery where life began. Their battle to climb the ladder defies explanation. I struggle to pull myself away when it's time to leave. Such tenacity, such persistence.

We are on the last leg of our cruise, sailing south along the west coast to Vancouver where we'll catch our flight home on July 25. A quick check of my calendar reminds me I have an appointment for my next scan on July 27, and another with Dr. McCart on July 31, in Toronto. It's going to be a busy week.

Sid steps in from the balcony, cell phone in hand.

"You can add an appointment for me. I just got a call from Dr. Robinson's office. She wants to see me on the 29th."

He had a check-up and some blood work the week before we left. I can see he's concerned. Something minor, I'm sure.

Another shock is delivered at our meeting with Dr. Robinson. She tells us that Sid's white blood count is abnormally high, and additional testing confirms he has early stage chronic lymphocytic leukemia (CLL). The good news, she is quick to reassure, is that it progresses very slowly and is treatable, so he should still count on dying of old age. He will see a specialist in September, Dr. John Matthews, Oncologist/Hematologist, at the Cancer Centre. Our emotions run the gamut. Being told you have cancer is never easy to hear, but learning it's considered manageable offers calming relief.

On the last day of July, we are back in Toronto for my appointment with Dr. McCart. I'm pleased to report my digestive tract continues to move slowly toward normalcy. My only complaint is an ongoing problem of hematuria, which I began to notice only a few weeks after my operation. Dr. Robinson has treated me for a couple of UTIs, but blood is still noticeable. Dr. McCart advises she will arrange for me to see a urologist, and once again, she delivers the glad tidings that my scan shows nothing of concern.

August is a busy month. Adam and family join us at the park for several days of camping, after which the boys stay on while Mom and Dad return home for work. Last year, Adam stayed to help because I was recovering from chemotherapy, but this year, we think we're up to the challenge. Sam and Will have a wonderful time, and although both Sid and I require a couple of days to recover, I'm very pleased.

Packing at our apartment is underway. We are excited to be moving to a brand-new building in Napanee on August 31. No one can understand why we'd give up our prime waterfront view, but I'm looking forward to a fresh start where there's been no sickness and misery. I'm very proud of my contribution to our move. Over several weeks, I pack a lot of boxes, then after the movers do their work, Betty Ann and I unpack and organize most of our belongings in only a few days.

Sid and I check in at the King Edward Hotel in Toronto on Saturday, September 26, 2015, for another happy occasion. We are guests at the wedding of my great-niece Allison and her fiancé, Dan. I'm so thrilled to be here, to be a part of this happy celebration, particularly when I think about where I was at this time last year. I carry with me a strong desire to experience this wonderful day, not only for myself, but on behalf of my mother, Marjorie, Allison's great-grandmother, and my sister Evelyn, Allison's grandmother, both of whom would have treasured this occasion. My mother's gold ring, with three birthstones representing her daughters, Evelyn, Betty Ann and myself, glitters on my finger. Allison is wearing her grandmother Evelyn's pearl necklace, which complements her beautiful wedding gown. Life is indeed an enigma—the pain and sadness of loss mixed with the joy and anticipation of the future.

The result of my visit with urologist Dr. Jason Izard, who performed a cystoscopy, was that he found no abnormalities and no explanation for the hematuria. Strangely enough, after this procedure, no more blood. Another sigh of relief—all problems should end so simply.

I have the misfortune of catching a nasty cold in October that ends with several days of severe coughing, resulting in an incisional hernia. How I wish I'd been hugging a pillow while I coughed, but with over a year between me and surgery, I didn't think it necessary. Perhaps I'll need to have it repaired at some point, but for now, I'm content to wait and see just how much of an inconvenience it is.

My cold retreats in time for the next CT scan and follow-up with Dr. Biagi. This is my one-year scan. If this one is good, the next scan will be in six months instead of three. Once again, I'm blessed with a good result, and the buildup of anxiety in my body releases and slides away.

My sixty-sixth birthday in December is an extended family gathering with dinner at the Riverfront Pub in Napanee, and I'm ever so pleased to be celebrating in good health.

As Christmas 2015 approaches, Sid and I decorate with anticipation—the family will celebrate with us in our new home this year. I'm a little worried about how we'll manage, but with a simple plan and everyone working together, what could go wrong?

When we moved to Napanee in September, I was very proud of the progress I'd made in regaining my strength. Even though

I can simply take the elevator to the third floor, I always use the stairs unless carrying a load. Gradually, as fall fades and winter advances, the degree of difficulty slowly builds until I choose only the elevator. Something is wrong. A trip to the doctor results in a blood test that shows my B12 is below recommended levels. If a supplement is all it takes to get my energy back, I'm laughing!

Sid and I choose to have a quiet evening at home on Valentine's Day rather than rubbing elbows with the Cupid crowd. After a simple but satisfying dinner, we watch the season finale of Saving Hope, a popular TV medical drama filmed in Toronto at the fictional Hope-Zion Hospital. Dr. Charlie Harris has just learned he has a malignant brain tumour. He expresses his thoughts in a way so familiar:

"And this is how it happens. In an instant, everything you think you know changes. The ground shifts, then gives way, and suddenly you're falling, hoping to God there's someone there to catch you."

Everyone who receives a diagnosis that in all likelihood will lead to premature death feels what Charlie felt. Perhaps they aren't able to express their feelings so eloquently. Perhaps they aren't able to express them at all. Some patients prefer not to talk about their ailment and skirt the dreaded C-word with phrases like "this thing that I have." It's a journey unique to each traveler.

A Caribbean cruise in March diverts my thoughts from the upcoming scan. The warm, moist breezes caress my skin, the natural beauty of our island stops, Aruba, Bonaire, Grenada, Dominica, St. Thomas, and Bahamas delights my eyes, and the continuous roll of blue-green surf quiets my mind. On the flight home, I'm all smiles reliving the pleasure of the past ten days. The islands are indeed beautiful, but I wonder how many islanders would have access to specialized care in their time of need?

HESITANT HOPE

It's six long months since the last scan. My imagination runs wild while the scanner whirrs and chirps in its unfamiliar language. Is it recording the beastly beginnings of new tumour growth? Is my good fortune running out?

The scan shows nothing of concern.

We're canoeing in a shallow, protected bay searching for a missing treasure. The eerie brushing of seaweed against the hull breaks the silence as our paddles strain through the tangled webs. There it is! Six velvet-white swans—cob, pen, and four beautiful cygnets. The young ones are still dependent, yet they are old enough to sport adult plumage. It's early July, and no sign of the swan family had us worried. These intelligent creatures choose to safeguard their brood in nature's womb until they are able to cope on a lake rife with motorboats and jet skis. We sit quietly for a moment, admiring this splendid sight, then make a slow retreat, giving them the privacy they deserve. These are awe-inspiring moments—moments that cradle the joys of life. It is good to be alive!

The ringing of my cell phone breaks into our conversation as Sid and I enjoy morning coffee on our sun-drenched deck.

"Hi Mom, are you in town or at the park?"

"We're at the park."

"Hailey and I are coming out. I have something to tell you."

"That was Sandy," I report, still holding the phone. "She's coming out—says she has something to tell us."

"I don't like the sound of that."

"Nor do I. What are you thinking?"

Sid shrugs. "Your guess is as good as mine."

In less than half an hour, we are sharing hello hugs. I offer to make coffee, and everyone follows me inside.

"I don't want to do this," Sandy starts, in obvious distress.

"You don't want to do what?" I ask with concern, a coffee mug in each hand.

"I don't want to tell you …… I have breast cancer," she sobs.

Noooooo …… I'm not hearing this … it can't be true!

"Are you sure?"

"Yes. I had a biopsy last week. I have invasive ductal carcinoma."

My arms are around her … a hug hardly seems an adequate response … I need to make this go away!

Over her shoulder, I see Hailey standing alone, trying to be brave while tell-tale tears dampen her cheeks. I motion her to join us. Then Sid's arms are there, encircling his girls.

As summer 2016 passes, Sandy submits to a radical mastectomy—now a day surgery—to be followed by chemotherapy, eight treatments in all at two-week intervals. In early 2017, there will be radiation treatments as well. Thankfully, I'm finding my experience as a cancer patient is allowing me to exhibit a degree of calm—calm that wouldn't be possible had I not already walked this road. I'll be better able to support her without falling apart at every turn.

Anger is a fairly common response to a cancer diagnosis, and although I've been the exception to the rule, at least for my diagnosis and Sid's, anger is building. Statistics indicate that approximately forty percent of our population will be diagnosed with cancer in their lifetime, but in my little family, we are now at seventy-five percent. Do we have targets painted on our backs?

Our handsome feline companion, Max, is also having a tough summer. He became part of our family fifteen years ago when we rescued him from a five-month stay at the local animal shelter. He'd been delivered to the shelter, together with several

HESITANT HOPE

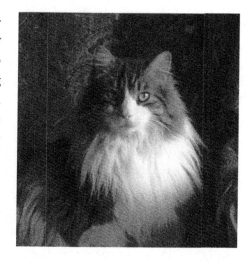

companions, the previous fall by a kindly rural matron who hated to see young barn kittens die of cold and starvation over the winter. Due to his surly disposition, however, he was not popular with those seeking to adopt until Sid and I decided he deserved a break. It took Max months to adapt to life as a house cat and to learn to trust us—to a degree. He never made a sound until he was about three years old, when he surprised us with a meow.

Max is sleeping more than usual and has little energy for play, although he's still keen to join me for my afternoon naps. By mid-August, his appetite is noticeably diminished, and he's too weak to jump into his favourite chair. Sid and I discuss the pros and cons of taking him to the veterinary clinic, but considering his age and the trauma the visit will inflict, we decide instead to keep a close watch on his quality of life. In only a few days, it's obvious his pleasure in living is gone. I place a call to a veterinarian who will come to our apartment so Max can be spared the upset of a clinic visit.

Max leaves us, cradled in Sid's arms, relaxed, watching me—as he's done so often—while I stroke his head and speak softly to him through my tears.

"You're such a good boy, Max. Thank you for all the help you gave me while I was sick."

How can I say good-bye to this amazing little creature who began life as a wild barn cat but cared enough to spend hours watching me, touching me, caring for me in his own special way during the stressful days of treatment and recovery? It may defy explanation, but I believe Max was an important part of my healing. Was that his way of thanking me for the life we gave him fifteen years ago?

The two-year anniversary of my surgery arrives on September 16, 2016. The next CT scan carries great significance. Most recurrences surface within the first two years, and I have reached that marker. Would I do it again? The answer is a resounding yes! No, I don't know what the upcoming scan will show, but I'm pleasingly healthy and happy at this time, whereas, had I not taken this treatment path, I'd be very ill by now. Yes, my normal *has* changed somewhat. There is still numbness in my hands and feet that causes fumbling and an unsteady gait. I occasionally experience pain in some joints and muscles that complained loudly at the beginning of each cycle of chemotherapy. To assist with declining energy levels and neuropathy, I'm receiving vitamin B12 by injection every two weeks to compensate for lack of absorption in my shortened intestinal tract. The lack of an insulating omentum means loud gurgling noises emanating from my belly, particularly when I bend. I've developed an incisional hernia and need to wear a brace when lifting. My memory and ability to concentrate suffered a significant blow. Of all the after-effects, this is the one that creates the most anxiety, and of course, anxiety makes it worse. It's frustrating when well-meaning people say, "Oh, it's just our age. I have the same problem." Try having twelve cycles of chemotherapy, then we'll talk. The phenomena called chemo brain is not well understood, and research is underway to study memory changes people with cancer experience.

When all is said and done, none of these symptoms are debilitating enough to take the joy out of living, and as time passes, I'm noticing small improvements in several areas, which hopefully will continue.

Then there's my scar. Most of the time I simply ignore it, but on occasion, when I'm foolish enough to stand naked in front of a mirror, I feel the need to express regret at how my body has been disfigured.

"You are beautiful, and your scar is beautiful," Sid insists. "That scar is the miracle that kept you with me."

THE END

EPILOGUE

My story will never really end. Cancer has a way of striking back, just when you think you're safe. I am happy to report, however, as of the date of publication, I am in good health.

GLOSSARY

Abdomen: That part of the trunk of the body lying between the thorax and the pelvis. It is separated from the thorax by the diaphragm.

Appendix: A small appendage near the juncture of the small intestine and the large intestine (ileocecal valve). An apparently useless structure, it can be the source of serious illness.

Arterial line: Thin catheter inserted into an artery, commonly used in intensive care medicine and anesthesia to monitor blood pressure, and to obtain samples for arterial gas analysis.

BMI: Body Mass Index (BMI). A number calculated from a person's weight and height which provides a reliable indicator of body fatness for most people.

Cautery: An agent or device used for scarring, burning, or cutting the skin or other tissues by means of heat, cold, electric current, ultrasound or caustic chemicals.

Cecum: The beginning of the large intestine and the place where the appendix attaches to the intestinal tract.

Chemo brain: A common term describing chemotherapy-related cognitive impairment or cognitive dysfunction.

Colon: The large intestine extending from the cecum to the rectum.

Cytoreductive surgery: Reducing the number of tumour cells by surgical means.

Diaphragm: Dome-shaped muscular partition separating the thorax from the abdomen.

Duodenum: The beginning portion of the small intestines, about 25 cm or 10 inches, starting at the lower end of the stomach.

ECG: An electrocardiogram is a tracing representing the heart's electrical action.

FOBT: Fecal occult blood test. It is used to detect microscopic blood in the stool.

Foley Catheter: Flexible tube passed through the urethra and into the bladder to drain urine.

HIPEC: Hyperthermic intraperitoneal chemotherapy. A highly concentrated, heated chemotherapy treatment that is delivered directly to the abdomen immediately following cytoreductive surgery in an attempt to kill the tumour cells that cannot be seen.

Hematuria: Blood in the urine.

Hemicolectomy: A colectomy procedure to remove one side of the colon is called a hemicolectomy. A right hemicolectomy involves removing the right side of the colon and attaching the small intestine to the remaining portion of the colon.

Hypoxemia: Abnormally low level of oxygen in the blood.

Intensivist: A physician who specializes in providing care to critically ill patients, especially those in an intensive care or coronary care unit.

Ileostomy: Surgical construction of an artificial excretory opening through the abdominal wall into the ileum.

Ileocecal valve: The sphincter muscle between the ileum of the small intestine and the cecum of the large intestine which prevents food from reentering the small intestine.

Ileum: The lower third of the small intestine, about 365 cm or 12 feet.

Laparoscopy: A type of surgical procedure in which a small incision is made through which a viewing tube (laparoscope) is inserted. The viewing tube has a small camera on the eyepiece.

This allows the doctor to examine the abdominal and pelvic organs on a video monitor connected to the tube.

Lesser omentum: Double layer of peritoneum that extends from the liver to the lesser curvature of the stomach and the first part of the duodenum.

Mitomycin-C: An anti-tumour antibiotic made from soil fungus. It inhibits DNA synthesis by producing DNA cross-links which halt cell replication and eventually cause cell death. Because cancer cells divide faster and with less error correcting than healthy cells, they are more sensitive to this damage.

Mucin: Gel or mucous-like substance normally produced by some organs to serve as lubrication. In the case of mucinous adenocarcinoma, this mucin is malignant in origin and if left untreated, will eventually build up, compressing abdominal organs.

NG tube: A tube used for suctioning stomach contents; inserted through the nose and down the esophagus into the stomach.

Nodule: Small collection of tissue that is palpable. Nodules characteristically range in size from 1 to 2 cm in diameter.

Omentum: A large apron of fatty tissue containing veins, arteries, lymphatic system. The omentum attaches to and nourishes the stomach and the entire colon.

Ostomy: Surgical procedure to create an opening (stoma) for waste to be released from the body into a bag. This can be a temporary or permanent procedure.

PCA: Patient-controlled analgesia is a drug-delivery system that dispenses a preset intravascular dose of a narcotic analgesic when the patient pushes a switch on an electric cord.

PMP Pals' Network: A support organization for those affected by Pseudomyxoma Peritonei (PMP), appendix cancer and other peritoneal surface disease.

Pelvis: The massive, cup-shaped ring of bone, with its ligaments, at the lower end of the trunk.

Peritoneum: A thin membrane that covers most abdominal organs and lines the abdominal cavity.
Pseudomyxoma Peritonei: A mucin-producing tumour of the appendix.
Resectable: Able to remove by surgery.
Spleen: Abdominal organ involved in the production and removal of blood cells, and forming part of the immune system.
Thorax: The part of the body between the neck and the abdomen.
Tumour: A mass of tissue caused by rapid cell division. These cells are uncontrollable and progressive. Tumours can be benign or malignant.
UTI: Urinary tract infection.

ACKNOWLEDGEMENTS

Although writing is a solitary endeavour, many people make important contributions.

My family played a crucial role in making my story complete. Thank you to my husband, Sid DeVries, my daughter, Sandy Johnson, and her husband, Geoff Johnson, and my son, Adam DeVries, all of whom were indispensable in providing additional details that I would not have been able to share without the benefit of their memories.

Maurice Breslow, fearless leader of the Wednesday afternoon writing workshop, together with my fellow students, gave valuable critique that kept me moving forward with confidence.

Both Dr. Andrea McCart and Dr. James Biagi found time to read the entire manuscript. They gave me the benefit of their medical expertise where needed, as well as providing encouraging comments.

I would also like to thank Pauline Barr, Betty Ann Bustard, Penny and Larry Dainard, Linda Veenstra, and Emma and Carman Willows for reading my second draft and providing their comments and encouragement.

The names of nursing staff and patients at Mount Sinai Hospital in Toronto have been changed.

CPSIA information can be obtained
at www.ICGtesting.com
Printed in the USA
LVOW03s0236080318
569054LV00001B/2/P